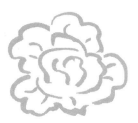

BONNIE SANDERS POLIN
AND FRANCES TOWNER GIEDT
WITH THE NUTRITION SERVICES STAFF
AT JOSLIN DIABETES CENTER

Other Books by These Authors

The Joslin Diabetes Gourmet Cookbook
The Joslin Diabetes Quick and Easy Cookbook

The Joslin Diabetes

Healthy Carbohydrate Cookbook

BONNIE SANDERS POLIN, PH.D.,
AND FRANCES TOWNER GIEDT

WITH THE NUTRITION SERVICES STAFF
AT THE JOSLIN DIABETES CENTER

Foreword by Alan C. Moses, M.D.,
Chief Medical Officer, Joslin Diabetes Center

A Fireside Book

PUBLISHED BY SIMON & SCHUSTER

New York • London • Toronto • Sydney • Singapore

FIRESIDE
Rockefeller Center
1230 Avenue of the Americas
New York, NY 10020

FIRESIDE and colophon are registered trademarks
of Simon & Schuster, Inc.

DESIGNED BY JILL WEBER

Manufactured in the United States of America
1   3   5   7   9   10   8   6   4   2

Library of Congress Cataloging-in-Publication Data

Polin, Bonnie Sanders, date.
The Joslin diabetes healthy carbohydrate cookbook / Bonnie Sanders Polin and
Frances Towner Giedt, with the Nutrition Services Staff at the Joslin Diabetes Center ;
foreword by Alan C. Moses
p.   cm.
Includes index.
1. Diabetes—Diet therapy—Recipes.   2. High-carbohydrate diet—Recipes.
I. Giedt, Frances Towner.   II. Joslin Diabetes Center.   III. Title.

RC662 .P632 2001
641.5'6314—dc21   00-053551
ISBN 0-684-86451-7

Acknowledgments

Producing a cookbook takes the talents of many hands and minds. We are lucky to have been able to surround ourselves with a network of knowledgeable people, so at the end of all our work we have another cookbook to be proud of.

We would like to thank

Our colleagues at the Joslin Diabetes Center and Joslin Clinic: Joan Hill, R.D., C.D.E., Director of Education; Karen Chalmers, M.S., R.D., C.D.E., Director of Nutrition; and the Nutrition and Diabetes Educators Judy Giusti, M.S., R.D., C.D.E.; Emmy Suhl, M.S., R.D., C.D.E.; Melinda Maryniuk, M. Ed., R.D., C.D.E., F.A.D.A.; Amy Campbell, M.S., R.D., C.D.E.; Maria Gallego, M.S., R.D., C.D.E.; Diana Hanson, R.D., and JoAnne Rizzotto, R.D., C.D.E. Our gratitude also to Susan Sjostrom, Director of Publications and Charlene Beal, Administrative Secretary. Your nutritional data for the recipes has helped us to create yet another invaluable cookbook for people with diabetes.

Our editors at Simon & Schuster, Becky Cabaza, Senior Editor, who worked with us on our first two diabetic cookbooks, for believing in this project; Marah Stets, Editor; Leslie Ellen, Copy Supervisor; Jill Weber, Book Designer; and Allyson Edelhertz, Editorial Assistant. For your insights, talents, and trust, we will always be grateful.

Our agent: Loretta Fidel for her diligence and guidance.

Finally, our husbands: Gerry Polin, M.D., and David Giedt for their constant encouragement, unending patience, or just a great night out away from the kitchen when we needed it.

—Bonnie Sanders Polin, Ph.D., and Frances Towner Giedt

This book is dedicated to the millions of people with diabetes who work hard each day to control this chronic disease so they may enjoy everyday life . . . and to the dedicated medical researchers around the world who continue to work tirelessly to make it easier for others to cope with diabetes, and to find the final cure.

Contents

The Joslin Diabetes

Healthy Carbohydrate Cookbook

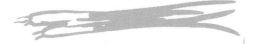

Foreword

*F*ood! Have you noticed how preoccupied we are with food? It is the center of most of our celebrations and the subject of countless advertisements that bombard us each day. Nutritional value, appearance, taste, fat content, carbohydrate content, and calories are just a few of the criteria we all use to evaluate food. For people who have diabetes, this list is longer and more complicated, perhaps even burdensome. Necessary regimentation, routine, scheduling, and the like can transform the joy and spontaneity of eating into "treatment" for diabetes. That's where *The Joslin Healthy Carbohydrate Cookbook* can help.

The recipes and tips in this book can help those with diabetes prepare foods that will not only enhance the joy of eating but also help in achieving good control of blood glucose levels. *The Joslin Healthy Carbohydrate Cookbook* also stresses the "heart healthy" nature of meal planning to help anyone with diabetes live a longer and healthier life.

During the last decade, major changes in the approach to dietary "treatment" of diabetes have occurred. The "routine" American Diabetes Association diet prescription as a standard has disappeared. Today meal planning should match individual treatment goals and the lifestyle of an individual patient. Using the simple guideline of "eating healthy," people who have diabetes currently have many more options and opportunities to succeed!

The Joslin Healthy Carbohydrate Cookbook has something for everyone, toddler to octogenarian. Frances Giedt and Bonnie Polin, along with the Joslin Clinic dietitians Judy Giusti and Joan Hill, have compiled a wide variety of recipes. Patients who want to reduce their total calories to lose weight will find many helpful hints in the pages of this book. In addition, patients on intensive diabetes treatment programs who need a better understanding of the exact carbohydrate content of foods in order to control their blood sugar levels within a range will find information at the end of each recipe.

The treatment of diabetes can seem both complicated and regimented to patients who lack experience or motivation in developing strategies to achieve their desired goals. A meal plan and exercise program are integral steps in this process. Use *The Joslin Healthy Carbohydrate Cookbook* as a source of ideas and support on this road to achieving treatment goals. It provides information, variety, and over 175 interesting and healthy recipes that will add to everyone's health and joy of eating!

Alan C. Moses, M.D., Chief Medical Officer
Joslin Diabetes Center and Joslin Clinic

Introduction

The relationship between food and its impact on diabetes management has dramatically changed over recent years. This has modified the way we eat and teach. First, our meal plans today are individualized. Carbohydrates may be high, protein moderate, and fat low in any given day. Second, our meal plan food choices are more varied, incorporating a myriad of foods, spices, and herbs from around the world, many unknown or unavailable to us until recent years. Nutrient distribution may vary depending on management tools. Home blood glucose monitoring, insulin flexibility, and exercise all impact one's meal plan approach.

Between us we have lived with diabetes for more than thirty years. As the authors of three cookbooks for people with diabetes, we have lectured to thousands, run a free diabetes clinic for the working poor, and currently publish an Internet monthly magazine about living with diabetes, *www.diabetic-lifestyle.com*. Millions of people in more than twenty-five countries read our magazine. We know the long-term complications that may be caused by not keeping blood glucose levels in target range. We also know the value of eating fresh vegetables, fruits, and other high-fiber foods to protect against other diseases such as cancer, heart disease, high blood pressure, kidney disease, and obesity.

Controlling Diabetes with Carbohydrates

When we lecture, the questions that arise most often are "Can one dine well on a diet of mostly carbohydrates?" and "Will a plant-based diet help me achieve good blood glucose control?" Our answer to both questions is a resounding "Yes." Carbohydrate-containing foods assume a significant part in diabetes meal planning, providing both carbohydrates and protein (as in dried beans, lentils, and other legumes and in tempeh and other forms of tofu). Using carbohydrate counting makes improved glycemic control possible, whether you are controlling diabetes by nutrition, insulin therapy, or oral medication. Work with your diabetes team to develop a meal plan approach that best suits your individual goals. We encourage you to use home blood glucose monitoring to fine-tune your treatment plan.

CARBOHYDRATE COUNTING

Carbohydrate counting is an easy way to keep track of the grams of carbohydrates (carbs) you eat at meals and snacks. Since almost all the carbohydrates you eat turn into glucose, you might imagine that eating the same amount of carbohydrates at each meal would make blood glucose more consistent. To simplify carbohydrate counting, round the value of milk up to 15 grams and count 1 fruit choice, 1 bread/starch choice, or 1 milk choice as 1 carbohydrate (carb) choice. Since nonstarchy vegetable choices usually contain 5 grams of carbohydrate, they are counted as vegetables unless consumed in sufficient quantity to contain 15 grams of carbohydrates, at which point they also become 1 carb choice. Carbohydrate flexibility comes into play for people who wish to adjust their insulin or exercise. Some people learn either sliding scales or carb-to-insulin ratios. Ask your diabetes team if this approach would improve your control.

ESTIMATING PORTION SIZE

In your own kitchen it's easy to measure portions using your scale and measuring cups and spoons. But it's also easy to estimate portion sizes by using the size of an average woman's hand (men may need to estimate down a little bit). A closed fist is about the size of 1 cup. Therefore, a fist-size portion of pasta or potato would be equal to 2 carbs (½ cup cooked pasta or potato equals 1 carbohydrate choice). One fist-size portion of cooked rice would be equal to 3 carbs (⅓ cup cooked rice equals 1 carbohydrate choice). A fist-size portion of strawberries would be equal to 1 carb (1 cup strawberries equals 1 carb choice). Look at the Joslin Diabetes Food Lists (page 233) to determine other portion sizes.

Your thumb is about 1 ounce of cheese or 1 tablespoon of salad dressing or peanut butter. Your thumb tip is about 1 teaspoon—use this for determining the size of fats, such as butter, margarine, mayonnaise, or oil.

PUTTING MEALS TOGETHER

Our meals are often composed of the tastes of many small dishes instead of a main dish, following the example of Chinese *dim sum,* Spanish *tapas,* or Mediterranean *mezze.* Other times we focus on a light main dish such as a vegetable stir-fry or dried bean stew, finding this to be eminently satisfying. Always we vary the textures and flavors, seldom repeating the same meal within a given week or month. To illustrate how easy it is to eat this way, there are sample menus starting on page 225.

In this cookbook we share some of our favorite recipes, which can be the basis of a vegetarian meal plan or, as they are for us, a good way to cut down on the saturated fats found in animal protein. You will note that most of the time we call for fresh foods rather than frozen or canned. We firmly believe that the end result is only as good as the ingredients that we use. We prefer to use fresh foods that we purchase locally because the taste of freshly picked produce is unequaled. Since we live in the jet age, this means that the best of the world is as close as our local supermarket—a luscious pineapple may have been picked on the big island of Hawaii just the day before. Farmer's markets offer the best of local crops, and our stores provide a wide variety of legumes, dried beans, and grains from around the world, so that our meals need never be dull. We do our part by growing fresh herbs in large pots by our kitchen doors and knowing where to find seedlings for the many varieties of basil, thyme, and other herbs that make our recipes sing.

A Healthy Carbohydrate Pantry

We both keep a well-stocked pantry so that making a meal does not mean running to the market every day. We market twice a week for fresh produce and then prepare our daily recipes using the staples in our pantry. Think small and keep your pantry inventory turning. Spices lose their aroma and flavor, oil loses its freshness, vinegar turns cloudy, and so on.

Cooking healthy meals that the entire family will enjoy becomes easy if you are not caught without an important ingredient just as your family or friends are ready to be seated for a meal. We also suggest that you invest in good-quality sharp knives and the best pots, pans, and kitchen tools you can afford. In the end, a well-stocked pantry and a top-notch selection of cooking tools will make your time in the kitchen easier and more pleasant. Here are some suggestions for stocking your pantry.

Vinegars

BALSAMIC

FRUIT-INFUSED

HERB-INFUSED

RED WINE

WHITE WINE

SHERRY

MALT

RICE WINE

CIDER

Cooking Sprays

BUTTER-FLAVORED

OLIVE OIL

VEGETABLE

Oils

CANOLA

OLIVE

PEANUT

SAFFLOWER

DARK SESAME

Grains

STONE-GROUND YELLOW AND WHITE
   CORNMEAL

COUSCOUS (QUICK-COOKING)

KASHA

MILLET

POLENTA (INSTANT)

QUINOA

RICE—WHITE, BASMATI, BROWN,
   AND WILD

ROLLED OATS

Beans and Legumes

DRIED BEANS—BLACK, CANNELLINI,
   CHICKPEAS, NAVY, PINTO, AND
   WHITE

LEGUMES—BROWN AND RED
   LENTILS, BLACK-EYED PEAS

Pasta

ANGEL HAIR

BOW-TIES (FARFALLE)

LINGUINE

PENNE

ASIAN RICE STICKS

ROTELLE

SPAGHETTI

ZITI

Baking Needs

UNBLEACHED ALL-PURPOSE FLOUR

NONFAT PANCAKE MIX

GRAHAM CRACKER CRUMBS

CORNSTARCH

DRY BREAD CRUMBS
   (UNSEASONED)

BAKING POWDER

BAKING SODA

CREAM OF TARTAR

COCOA POWDER

REGULAR AND KOSHER SALT

VANILLA EXTRACT

ARTIFICIAL SWEETENERS
   (CAPABLE OF RETAINING SWEET-
   NESS DURING EXTENDED HEAT)

GRANULATED SUGAR

BROWN SUGAR

BAKER'S SPRAY (COMBINED WITH
   FLOUR)

Canned and Packaged Goods

NO-SALT-ADDED TOMATO PASTE

NO-SALT-ADDED CANNED TOMATOES

CANNED LOW-FAT, LOW-SODIUM
   CHICKEN AND VEGETABLE
   BROTH

REDUCED-SODIUM SOY SAUCE

NO-SUGAR-ADDED FRUIT SPREAD

DRY-ROASTED PEANUTS

NATURAL PEANUT BUTTER

NO-SUGAR-ADDED DRIED FRUITS

EVAPORATED SKIM MILK

POWDERED BUTTERMILK

WORCESTERSHIRE SAUCE

HOT PEPPER SAUCE

DIJON MUSTARD—REGULAR AND
   COARSE-GROUND

DRY RED AND WHITE WINE

COGNAC

HOISIN SAUCE

SUN-DRIED TOMATOES
(DRY-PACKED)

BLACK BEAN SAUCE

ASIAN CHILI SAUCE

CAPERS

GARLIC SAUCE

DRIED CHILES

DRIED MUSHROOMS

Dried Herbs and Spices

GROUND ALLSPICE

BASIL

BAY LEAVES

CARAWAY SEED

CELERY SEED

CHILI POWDER

GROUND CINNAMON

CLOVES—WHOLE AND GROUND

CORIANDER—SEED AND GROUND

CUMIN—SEED AND GROUND

CURRY POWDER

DILL

FENNEL SEED

FINES HERBES

GROUND GINGER

MARJORAM

DRY MUSTARD

PAPRIKA

PEPPERCORNS

POPPY SEEDS

CRUSHED RED PEPPER FLAKES

ROSEMARY

SAGE

SAFFRON

SAVORY

SESAME SEEDS

THYME

In the Freezer

FROZEN NO-SUGAR-ADDED FRUITS
AND BERRIES

PUFF PASTRY DOUGH

FILO DOUGH

BREAD DOUGH

REDUCED-CALORIE MARGARINE

NUTS

VEGETABLES IN BAGS

MULTIGRAIN BREADS AND ROLLS

In the Refrigerator

PART-SKIM PARMESAN CHEESE

LOW-FAT AND FAT-FREE
MOZZARELLA CHEESE

LOW-FAT AND FAT-FREE RICOTTA
CHEESE

LOW-FAT AND FAT-FREE CREAM
CHEESE

REDUCED-FAT TUB MARGARINE

FAT-FREE SOUR CREAM

FRESH GINGER

LEMONS

LIMES

ORANGES

OTHER FRESH FRUIT IN SEASON

SCALLIONS

FRESH HERBS AND PARSLEY

SALAD INGREDIENTS

FRESH VEGETABLES IN SEASON

DILL PICKLES

TOMATO PASTE IN A TUBE

ANCHOVY PASTE IN A TUBE

EGG SUBSTITUTE

EGGS

SKIM MILK

Miscellaneous

GARLIC

ONIONS

POTATOES

SWEET POTATOES

SHALLOTS

The Joslin Diabetes Center

Once again, we thank our colleagues at Joslin Diabetes Center and the Joslin Clinic, affiliated with Harvard Medical School, for their help and expertise. We are proud to be associated with the staff of this eminent facility, which leads the medical community in the research and treatment of diabetes. We continue to look to it for breakthroughs that will help us all in the control and final cure of diabetes. Joslin is the oldest free-standing institution in the United States dedicated solely to diabetes. Joslin offers numerous publications, including *The Joslin Guide to Diabetes: A Program for Managing Your Treatment* (a Fireside book published by Simon & Schuster), by Richard A. Beaser, M.D., with Joan V. C. Hill, R.D., C.D.E. New at Joslin's Web site, www.joslin.org, is a chat room monitored by a registered dietitian, a social worker, and a diabetes educator, who will address your questions about nutrition and diabetes issues.

Nutritional Information

Our recipes were calculated by Judy Giusti, M.S., R.D., C.D.E., of the Joslin Diabetes Center's Nutrition Services. Joslin Choices and nutritional information are listed for each recipe using the latest data available from ESHA (*The Food Processor,* Version 7.3); the United States Department of Agriculture; and, when necessary, manufacturers' food labels.

Appetizers and Quick Snacks

Bruschetta

*B*ruschetta is the original garlic toast and one of Italy's simplest feasts. Grilled bread is rubbed with fresh garlic, then topped with fresh herbs, grilled vegetables, cheese, or almost any savory dip or spread. Bruschetta makes a wonderful snack when made a few pieces at a time, an easy appetizer when you make more, or elegant hors d'oeuvres for a party. The toasts are also terrific to serve with salads and soups as a crisp accompaniment.

1 narrow Italian, French, or sourdough bread (about 1 pound), sliced ½ inch thick
olive oil cooking spray
cut cloves of garlic

Grill or toast the bread slices until browned on both sides. While still warm, spray with cooking spray. Rub with a cut clove of garlic.

Makes 10 pieces.

JOSLIN CHOICES: 1½ carbohydrate (bread/starch)
PER SERVING: 127 calories (10% calories from fat), 1 g total fat (0 saturated fat), 4 g protein, 24 g carbohydrates, 1 g dietary fiber, 0 cholesterol, 276 mg sodium, 57 mg potassium

Toppings for Bruschetta

*W*e suggest a gutsy combination of arugula, roasted tomato, and low-fat cheese; Baba Ghanoush (a fabulous smoky eggplant dip that we love); shiitake mushrooms with low-fat feta cheese; a spicy tomato topping; grilled summer squash with a splash of aged balsamic vinegar; and white beans with a lively combination of Tuscan flavors. You could also use hummus (page 33).

Arugula, Roasted Tomato, and Goat Cheese

2 large tomatoes, roasted (page 202)
1 large bunch arugula, well washed, dried, and coarsely chopped (about 2 cups)
1 tablespoon olive oil
16 bruschetta (page 21)
4 ounces low-fat goat cheese

Peel, seed, and chop the tomatoes. Place in a bowl and combine with the arugula. Drizzle with the olive oil and toss to coat evenly.

When ready to serve, spread each bruschetta with ½ tablespoon goat cheese. Top with 2 tablespoons of the tomato-arugula mixture. Serve at once.

Makes 16 pieces.

JOSLIN CHOICES: 2 carbohydrate (bread/starch)
PER I-BRUSCHETTA SERVING: 172 calories (21% calories from fat), 4 g total fat (2 g saturated fat), 6 g protein, 25 carbohydrates, 1 g dietary fiber, 7 mg cholesterol, 303 mg sodium, 120 mg potassium.
PER SERVING (TOPPING ONLY): 45 calories (68% calories from fat), 3 g total fat (2 g saturated fat), 2 g protein, 1 g carbohydrates, 0 dietary fiber, 7 mg cholesterol, 27 mg sodium, 63 mg potassium

Baba Ghanoush

1 large eggplant (about 1 pound)
2 large cloves garlic, minced
juice of 1 large lemon
2 tablespoons tahini
2 tablespoons water
1 tablespoon olive oil
2 tablespoons chopped fresh cilantro
⅛ teaspoon kosher salt (optional)
freshly ground pepper to taste
bruschetta (page 21)
flat-leaf parsley sprigs

Preheat the oven to 425°F.

Prick the eggplant with a fork in several places and place on a baking sheet. Bake until very soft and the skin chars and shrivels, about 30 minutes. Remove from the oven and allow to cool to the touch.

Peel the eggplant and finely chop the flesh. Place in a bowl with the garlic, lemon juice, tahini, water, olive oil, cilantro, salt (if using), and pepper. Chill for at least 2 hours to allow the flavors to blend.

To serve, place 2 teaspoons on each piece of bruschetta and garnish with a sprig of parsley.

Makes about 1¼ cups, enough for 30 bruschetta.

JOSLIN CHOICES: 1½ carbohydrate (bread/starch)
PER 1-BRUSCHETTA SERVING: 142 calories (12% calories from fat), 2 g total fat (0 saturated
   fat), 4 g protein, 25 g carbohydrates, 1 g dietary fiber, 0 cholesterol, 285 mg sodium, 100
   mg potassium

Mushrooms with Feta Cheese

olive oil cooking spray
1 tablespoon olive oil
2 large cloves garlic, minced
4 ounces fresh shiitake mushrooms, cleaned, stemmed, and coarsely chopped
3 tablespoons dry white wine
3 tablespoons fresh lemon juice
1 teaspoon minced fresh thyme or ¼ teaspoon crushed dried
½ teaspoon minced fresh rosemary or ⅛ teaspoon crushed dried
¼ teaspoon salt (optional)
freshly ground pepper to taste
12 bruschetta (page 21)
2 ounces low-fat feta cheese, crumbled
¼ cup chopped flat-leaf parsley

Lightly coat a nonstick skillet with cooking spray. Add the olive oil and place over medium heat. Add the garlic and cook, stirring, until it is golden (be careful not to burn). Using a slotted spoon, transfer the garlic to a paper towel. Set aside.

Again spray the skillet with cooking spray. Add the mushrooms and cook over medium-high heat, stirring, until they wilt, about 5 minutes. Add the wine and lemon juice. Cook, stirring, until the liquid is absorbed. Stir in the thyme, rosemary, salt (if using), and pepper.

To serve, divide the mushroom mixture among the bruschetta as a topping. Sprinkle each with ½ tablespoon crumbled feta cheese and some parsley. Serve at once.

Makes 12 pieces

JOSLIN CHOICES: 2 carbohydrate (bread/starch)

PER I-BRUSCHETTA SERVING: 161 calories (17% calories from fat), 3 g total fat (1 g saturated fat), 6 g protein, 26 g carbohydrates, 1 g dietary fiber, 3 mg cholesterol, 351 mg sodium, 90 mg potassium

PER SERVING (TOPPING ONLY): 34 calories (51% calories from fat), 2 g total fat (1 g saturated fat), 2 g protein, 2 g carbohydrates, 0 dietary fiber, 3 mg cholesterol, 75 mg sodium, 33 mg potassium

Mexican Tomato Relish

2 large ripe tomatoes (about 1 pound total), finely chopped
½ red onion (3 ounces), minced
2 large cloves garlic, minced
1 jalapeño chile pepper, seeded and finely minced
2 tablespoons lime juice
3 tablespoons chopped fresh cilantro, plus extra for garnish
bruschetta (page 21)

In a bowl, combine the tomatoes, onion, garlic, jalapeño, lime juice, and cilantro. Allow to sit at room temperature for 1 hour before serving.

To serve, place 2 tablespoons of the relish on each piece of bruschetta. Garnish with extra cilantro.

Makes about 2 cups, enough for 16 bruschetta.

JOSLIN CHOICES: 1½ carbohydrate (bread/starch)

PER 1-BRUSCHETTA SERVING: 137 calories (7% calories from fat), 1 g total fat (0 saturated fat), 4 g protein, 26 g carbohydrates, 0 dietary fiber, 0 cholesterol, 279 mg sodium, 135 mg potassium

PER SERVING (TOPPING ONLY): 10 calories (10% calories from fat), 0 total fat (0 saturated fat), 4 g protein, 26 g carbohydrates, 0 dietary fiber, 0 cholesterol, 3 mg sodium, 78 mg potassium

Grilled Summer Squash with Balsamic Splash

½ pound summer squash, sliced ½ inch thick on the diagonal
olive oil cooking spray
1 tablespoon balsamic vinegar
1 tablespoon grated Parmesan cheese
8 bruschetta (page 21)

Light a grill or preheat the broiler.

Lightly coat the squash slices with cooking spray and place on the grill or under the broiler. Sprinkle with the vinegar. Grill or broil on one side until browned. Turn and spray again with cooking spray. Sprinkle with the cheese. Cook 1 minute more. Place 1 slice on each piece of bruschetta and serve.

Makes 8 bruschetta.

JOSLIN CHOICES: 1½ carbohydrate (bread/starch)
PER 1-BRUSCHETTA SERVING: 137 calories (7% calories from fat), 1 g total fat (0 g saturated fat), 5 g protein, 26 g carbohydrates, 1 g dietary fiber, 1 mg cholesterol, 291 mg sodium, 114 mg potassium

PER SERVING (TOPPING ONLY): 10 calories (26% calories from fat), 0 total fat (0 saturated fat), 1 g protein, 2 g carbohydrates, 0 dietary fiber, 1 mg cholesterol, 15 mg sodium, 57 mg potassium

Tuscan White Beans

1 15-ounce can cannellini beans, rinsed and well drained
1 large plum tomato, seeded and minced

1 small onion, finely minced
1 large clove garlic, finely minced
4 to 5 fresh sage leaves, minced, or ½ teaspoon crushed dried
1 tablespoon olive oil
bruschetta (page 21)
freshly ground pepper to taste
chopped fresh basil or flat-leaf parsley

In a bowl, combine the beans, tomato, onion, garlic, and sage. Drizzle with the olive oil and toss to coat evenly. Allow to sit at room temperature for 30 minutes to allow the flavors to blend.

To serve, spoon 2 tablespoons of the bean mixture on a bruschetta. Grind pepper over the topping and sprinkle with basil. Serve at once.

Makes about 2 cups, enough for 16 bruschetta.

JOSLIN CHOICES: 2 carbohydrate (bread/starch)
PER 1-BRUSCHETTA SERVING: 160 calories (11% calories from fat), 2 g total fat (0 saturated
    fat), 5 g protein, 29 g carbohydrates, 2 g dietary fiber, 0 cholesterol, 329 mg sodium, 79 mg
    potassium
PER SERVING (TOPPING ONLY): 33 calories (27% calories from fat), 1 g total fat
    (0 saturated fat), 1 g protein, 5 g carbohydrates, 1 g dietary fiber, 0 cholesterol, 56 mg
    sodium, 22 mg potassium

Dried Herbs

Crush dried herbs in the palm of your hand before adding to a dish to release their volatile oils. Dried herbs quickly lose their flavor when exposed to heat and light. When in doubt, sniff. If the aroma isn't there, the flavor won't be either. Be prudent when using dried herbs when the recipe calls for fresh. Usually one-third of the amount called for fresh is the key, but your taste buds must make the final decision.

Baked Pita Chips

*W*e find so many uses for these delicious chips that we make them in big batches, storing them in a self-sealing plastic bag. Serve them with dips and spreads, with salads, or alone as a quick snack. Recently we discovered a can of fire-roasted garlic juice that you can spritz onto the pita triangles just prior to baking. Look for the garlic juice in specialty foods store and mail-order food catalogs.

> *6 6-inch pita breads*
> *olive oil cooking spray*
> *fire-roasted garlic juice (optional)*

Preheat the oven to 375°F.

With a sharp knife, cut each pita bread in half, then cut each half into 3 triangles. Gently pull apart each triangle to separate it into 2 pieces, getting 12 triangles per pita bread.

Lay the triangles in a single layer on a large nonstick baking sheet. (Depending on the size of your baking sheet, you may need to bake them in 2 batches.) Lightly coat the triangles with cooking spray and spritz lightly with garlic juice (if using). Bake for about 7 minutes, until the pitas begin to color. Turn them over and continue to bake until crisp and golden brown, about another 5 minutes. Store in airtight containers or self-sealing plastic bags.

Makes 72 pita chips.

VARIATIONS:

You can vary these pita chips according to the use and flavor that you prefer. Try one of the following ingredients sprinkled on the chips before baking: fennel or anise seeds, crushed red pepper flakes, curry powder and spices, or finely chopped fresh herbs of your choice.

JOSLIN CHOICES: I carbohydrate (bread/starch)

PER 6-CHIP SERVING: 83 calories (4% calories from fat), 0 total fat (0 saturated fat), 3 g protein, 17 g carbohydrates, I g dietary fiber, 0 cholesterol, 161 mg sodium, 36 mg potassium

Spicy Lentil Dip

*L*entils have a subtle savor that melds with other ingredients to make a pleasing, spicy dip. We use pink or red lentils for their color. If you purchase your lentils at an Indian market, you may find *massar dal,* or pink lentils. In other markets you'll likely find only red lentils.

> *1 pound dried pink or red lentils, rinsed and picked over*
> *6 cups water*
> *1 large head garlic (about 12 cloves), roasted*
> *1 red serrano chile pepper, seeded and finely minced*
> *1½ tablespoons fresh lemon juice*
> *1 tablespoon olive oil*
> *1 teaspoon ground cumin*
> *salt to taste (optional)*
> *freshly ground pepper to taste*
> *2 tablespoons minced flat-leaf parsley*

Place the lentils and water in a large saucepan. Bring to a boil; reduce the heat to simmer. Cook, stirring occasionally, until the lentils are very soft, about 35 to 45 minutes. Drain in a fine-mesh sieve.

Transfer the lentils to a food processor fitted with a metal blade. Separate the garlic cloves and squeeze the roasted garlic pulp into the work bowl. Add the chile pepper, lemon juice, olive oil, cumin, salt (if using), and pepper. Process until smooth. Transfer the mixture to a serving bowl and sprinkle parsley around the outside edge. Serve with Baked Pita Chips (page 27) or crudités.

Makes 4 cups.

JOSLIN CHOICES: 1 very-low-fat protein, ½ carbohydrate (bread/starch)
PER ¼-CUP SERVING (DIP ONLY): 109 calories (9% calories from fat), 1 g total fat
    (0 saturated fat), 8 g protein, 17 g carbohydrates, 9 g dietary fiber, 0 cholesterol, 4 mg
    sodium, 282 mg potassium

Seasoned Bean Dip

*S*everal upscale restaurants serve a version of this well-seasoned dip. Ours is based on one we sampled at Union Square Café in Manhattan, where it was served with baked pita chips as a light appetizer. It's also excellent with assorted crudités.

olive oil cooking spray
2 shallots, finely chopped
1 large clove garlic, minced
½ tablespoon ground cumin
⅛ to ¼ teaspoon crushed dried red chiles
1 15-ounce can white beans, such as cannellini, rinsed and drained
¼ cup grated Monterey Jack cheese (about 1 ounce)
¼ cup plain nonfat yogurt
¼ tablespoon fresh lemon juice
cayenne pepper to taste

Lightly coat a heavy nonstick skillet with cooking spray. Place over medium-low heat and add the shallots and garlic. Cook, stirring often, until the vegetables are limp but not browned, about 4 minutes. Add the cumin and crushed dried chiles. Cook, stirring, for 1 minute. Add the beans and continue to cook for another 3 to 4 minutes, stirring constantly.

Transfer the hot mixture to a food processor fitted with a metal blade. Add the cheese, yogurt, and lemon juice. Process until smooth. Transfer the mixture to a serving bowl. Sprinkle with cayenne. Serve at once or cover and refrigerate for up to 1 day.

Makes about 2 cups.

JOSLIN CHOICES: ½ low-fat protein, 1 carbohydrate (bread/starch)
PER ½-CUP SERVING (DIP ONLY): 139 calories (20% calories from fat), 3 g total fat (2 g
    saturated fat), 7 g protein, 20 g carbohydrates, 5 g dietary fiber, 7 mg cholesterol, 274 mg
    sodium, 131 mg potassium

~STUFFED VEGETABLES~

*S*tuffing vegetables with savory herbs and cheese changes them from ho-hum to something special. You'll note that some of the stuffings here can be used as dips. All of the stuffed vegetables make perfect little vegetable appetizers; some make wonderful side-dish accompaniments to a meal.

Belgian Endive with Herbed Ricotta

*B*elgian endive is best soaked in ice water before serving. Merely remove one leaf at a time and place in the water. The combination of the sweet cheese mixture against the crisp, tangy endive makes a light and appealing appetizer. This is particularly stunning if your market offers red Belgian endive. You could also use tiny leaves of radicchio.

> *¾ cup low-fat ricotta cheese*
> *2 tablespoons fresh lemon juice*
> *3 tablespoons chopped fresh flat-leaf parsley*
> *1 small clove garlic, minced*
> *1½ tablespoons chopped fresh chives*
> *1 tablespoon chopped fresh tarragon or 1 teaspoon crushed dried*
> *1 scallion, white part and 1 inch green, minced*
> *freshly ground pepper to taste*
> *16 Belgian endive leaves, soaked in ice water and dried*
> *extra parsley or tarragon for garnish*

In the bowl of a food processor fitted with the metal blade, place the ricotta, lemon juice, parsley, garlic, chives, tarragon, scallion, and pepper. Blend until smooth.

Place 1 tablespoon of the cheese mixture on the stem end of the endive leaf. Arrange on a platter and garnish with parsley or tarragon.

Makes 4 servings.

JOSLIN CHOICES: ½ low-fat protein, I vegetable

PER SERVING: 80 calories (41% calories from fat), 4 g total fat (2 g saturated fat), 6 g protein,
6 g carbohydrates, 2 g dietary fiber, 14 mg cholesterol, 73 mg sodium, 10 mg potassium

Mushrooms Stuffed with Garlic Mashed Potatoes

*T*hese are quite delicious and so easy to make. Serve them as a simple appetizer or snack or as part of an assorted cooked vegetable platter.

1 10-ounce russet potato, peeled and cut into quarters
2 large cloves garlic, peeled
2 tablespoons egg substitute
2 tablespoons skim milk
¼ teaspoon kosher salt (optional)
freshly ground pepper to taste
1 8-ounce package button mushrooms
butter-flavored cooking spray

Preheat the oven to 400°F.

Place the potatoes and garlic cloves in boiling water to cover and simmer for 15 to 20 minutes, until the potatoes are tender when pierced with the tip of a sharp knife and the garlic is very soft. Drain well and place in a bowl.

Mash or rice the potatoes and garlic. Add the egg substitute and milk, beating to a smooth texture. Season with salt (if using) and pepper.

Clean the mushrooms; remove and discard the stems. Drain briefly, stem side down, on paper towels. Fill each mushroom cap with 1 tablespoon of the garlic potatoes, mounding in the center. Place on a baking dish. Lightly coat each mushroom with cooking spray and bake for about 10 to 15 minutes, until the caps have softened and the potatoes begin to brown. Serve immediately.

Makes 16 to 20 stuffed mushrooms.

JOSLIN CHOICES (4 mushrooms): I carbohydrate (bread/starch), I vegetable

PER SERVING: 103 calories (5% calories from fat), I g total fat (0 saturated fat), 4 g protein,
21 g carbohydrates, 2 g dietary fiber, 0 cholesterol, 144 mg sodium, 551 mg potassium

Red Potato Nibbles

*T*hese little bites make a wonderful addition to a cold meal and shine as an appetizer or hors d'oeuvre. The easiest way to prepare the spinach base for this recipe is to roll a few leaves and then slice crosswise into very thin strips called chiffonade.

12 tiny new red potatoes (about 1 ounce each)
1 small carrot, grated
2 tablespoons chopped fresh dill
¼ cup finely chopped fresh baby spinach (about ½ ounce)
1 tablespoon white wine vinegar
2 tablespoons nonfat mayonnaise
2 tablespoons low-fat sour cream
⅛ teaspoon salt (optional)
freshly ground pepper to taste
extra spinach, cut in chiffonade, for serving

Place the potatoes in a pot of boiling water and cook about 15 minutes, or until tender. Drain and set aside until cool enough to handle.

Cut the potatoes in half and then cut a very thin slice from the bottom of each half so that they sit upright. With a small melon baller, remover the center of each half, being careful to leave a strong shell so that they do not break. Chop the potato balls that you have removed and place in a small bowl

Toss the potatoes with the carrot, dill, chopped spinach, vinegar, mayonnaise, sour cream, salt (if using), and pepper. Mound 2 teaspoons of the mixture onto each potato half. Refrigerate until ready to serve.

To serve, arrange the potatoes on a dish of chiffonade spinach.

Makes 6 servings.

JOSLIN CHOICES: 1 carbohydrate (bread/starch)
PER SERVING: 66 calories (7% calories from fat), 0 fat (0 saturated fat), 2 g protein, 14 g
    carbohydrates, 2 g dietary fiber, 2 mg cholesterol, 88 mg sodium, 261 mg potassium

Cherry Tomatoes Stuffed with Hummus

*H*ummus may also be served with pita bread and fresh vegetables for lunch or with baked pita chips as a dip. It makes a delicious topping for grilled vegetables or bruschetta. Keep this tasty Middle Eastern treat in your refrigerator; use within five days.

1 15-ounce can chickpeas, rinsed and drained well
1 clove garlic
2 tablespoons tahini
1 tablespoon olive oil
2 to 3 tablespoons fresh lemon juice
1 tablespoon water
½ teaspoon kosher salt (optional)
¼ teaspoon ground cumin
freshly ground pepper to taste
1 12-ounce package cherry tomatoes

Place the chickpeas in a food processor or blender. Add the garlic, tahini, olive oil, 2 tablespoons lemon juice, water, salt (if using), cumin, and pepper. Process until the hummus is smooth and has the consistency of heavy whipped cream. Add more lemon juice to taste.

Cut the tops off the cherry tomatoes and gently squeeze out the seeds. Place 1 teaspoon of hummus in each tomato and serve.

Makes about 32 to 36 stuffed tomatoes.

JOSLIN CHOICES (4 tomatoes): 1 carbohydrate (bread/starch), 1 fat
PER SERVING: 112 calories (36% calories from fat), 5 g total fat (1 g saturated fat), 4 g
protein, 15 g carbohydrates, 3 g dietary fiber, 0 cholesterol, 281 mg sodium, 208 mg
potassium

Baby Zucchini with Low-Fat Goat Cheese

*B*aby vegetables are easier to find in today's supermarkets, and these small zucchini make perfect hors d'oeuvres. We like to stuff them with a savory filling and top with a bit of fresh goat cheese.

> *4 small zucchini (about 1 pound total)*
> *olive oil cooking spray*
> *½ cup minced onion*
> *¼ cup bread crumbs*
> *¼ cup egg substitute*
> *½ teaspoon crushed dried fines herbes*
> *¼ teaspoon salt (optional)*
> *freshly ground pepper to taste*
> *4 teaspoons crumbled low-fat goat cheese*

Preheat the oven to 425°F.

Cut each zucchini in half lengthwise, leaving any blossoms on one of the halves. With the tip of a vegetable peeler or grapefruit spoon, carefully scoop out the pulp, making a ¼-inch-thick shell. Finely chop the flesh; set aside.

Lightly coat a nonstick skillet with cooking spray. Add the onion and chopped zucchini. Cook over medium heat until soft, about 5 minutes. Remove from the heat. Stir in the bread crumbs and combine well, then add the egg substitute, herbs, salt (if using), and pepper.

Stuff each zucchini shell with ⅛ of the stuffing. Sprinkle the cheese over the stuffing. Place on a baking sheet and spray each stuffed zucchini with cooking spray. Bake 15 to 25 minutes, until the zucchini shells soften but still hold their shape. Serve immediately, whole or cut into quarters for bite-size hors d'oeuvres.

Makes 4 servings.

JOSLIN CHOICES: I low-fat protein, 2 vegetable
PER SERVING: 96 calories (21% calories from fat), 2 g total fat (1 g saturated fat), 9 g protein,
I I g carbohydrates, 2 g dietary fiber, 3 mg cholesterol, 322 mg sodium, 628 mg potassium

Baked Egg Rolls with Mustard and Sweet and Hot Dipping Sauces

*B*aking these egg rolls makes them crispy and greaseless without taking away any of the gingery and garlicky taste we remember from our favorite Asian restaurants.

vegetable cooking spray
⅛ teaspoon dark sesame oil
½ cup egg substitute
1 3.2-ounce package fresh shiitake mushrooms, cleaned, stems removed, and thinly sliced
2 cups bean sprouts
2 cups shredded Napa cabbage
1½ tablespoons grated fresh ginger
1½ teaspoons minced garlic
1½ teaspoons cornstarch
1 tablespoon reduced-sodium soy sauce
2 tablespoons water
8 7-inch egg roll wrappers
1 egg white beaten with 1 tablespoon water

SWEET AND HOT DIPPING SAUCES
purchased Chinese mustard sauce (optional)
2 tablespoons prepared horseradish
2 tablespoons red wine vinegar
2 tablespoons reduced-sodium soy sauce
¼ teaspoon sugar substitute

Lightly coat a small nonstick sauté pan with cooking spray, then add the sesame oil. Place over medium heat and add the egg substitute. Cook until set, and then turn. Slide onto a plate and cool. Slice into thin 1-inch-long strips and set aside.

Lightly coat a nonstick skillet big enough for the vegetables and add the mushrooms, bean sprouts, cabbage, ginger, and garlic. Stir-fry over high heat for 2 minutes.

Combine the cornstarch, soy sauce, and water in a cup and pour over the vegetables. Stir-fry for another minute and then remove from the heat. Stir in the egg strips.

Lightly coat a heavy baking sheet with cooking spray.

To make the egg rolls, place a wrapper on a work surface with 1 corner facing you. Place ⅛ of the filling in the bottom third of the wrapper. Fold the bottom corner over the filling to cover, then roll over once to enclose filling. Fold over left and right corners, then brush the sides and top of the triangle with beaten egg white. Roll, sealing the corner. Place on the prepared baking sheet, folded side down. Cover while you fill the remaining wrappers. (May be made ahead to this point, covered, and refrigerated for up to 8 hours.)

Preheat the oven to 450°F.

To prepare the sauces, spoon some of the Chinese mustard sauce (if using) into a small serving bowl. In another small serving bowl, combine the horseradish, vinegar, soy sauce, and sugar substitute, mixing well.

Bake the egg rolls for 4 minutes, until the bottoms brown. Turn and bake 2 to 3 minutes more, until the underside is browned. Serve immediately with the dipping sauces.

Makes 8 egg rolls.

JOSLIN CHOICES (1 roll): 1 carbohydrate (bread/starch), 2 vegetable
PER SERVING: 135 calories (8% calories from fat), 1 g total fat (0 saturated fat), 7 g protein,
    24 g carbohydrates, 2 g dietary fiber, 3 mg cholesterol, 434 mg sodium, 208 mg potassium

Vietnamese Imperial Rolls with Peanut Dipping Sauce

Vietnamese food is becoming quite popular throughout much of the country. Based primarily on fresh vegetables and herbs, it's easy to prepare at home.

Here we've made Vietnamese Imperial Rolls, a variety of spring rolls, using rice paper wrappers that you can buy at some supermarkets, Asian food markets, and natural food stores. The wrappers will dry out if not eaten soon after they're made, so prepare the filling, lettuce, and sauce earlier in the day to allow the flavors to blend. Then soak and roll the rice paper rounds just before serving. They make a marvelous snack or savory beginning to a meal.

1½ ounces cellophane noodles
1 small carrot (2 ounces), grated
1 cup (2 ounces) bean sprouts
1 cup (2 ounces) shredded Napa cabbage
2 scallions, cut into 4 1-inch pieces, julienned
8 snow peas (½ ounce), stringed and julienned
juice of 1 small lime
3 tablespoons chopped fresh cilantro
2 tablespoons chopped fresh mint
1 large clove garlic, minced
⅛ to ¼ teaspoon crushed red pepper flakes, to taste
⅛ teaspoon sugar substitute

Dipping Sauce
1½ tablespoons red wine vinegar
1 tablespoon water
1 tablespoon reduced-sodium soy sauce
1 tablespoon creamy no-oil-added peanut butter
1 small clove garlic, minced
⅛ teaspoon sugar substitute
⅛ to ¼ teaspoon crushed red pepper flakes, to taste

8 large rice paper rounds (wrappers)
4 large leaves Boston lettuce, core removed, rinsed and dried

Cover the cellophane noodles with hot water and soak for 20 to 30 minutes, until softened. Drain and cut into 2-inch pieces.

Place the noodles in a bowl along with the carrot, bean sprouts, cabbage, scallions, and snow peas. In a cup, whisk the lime juice, cilantro, mint, garlic, red pepper flakes, and sugar substitute. Pour over the vegetable mixture; toss and set aside.

To prepare the dipping sauce, whisk together the vinegar, water, soy sauce, peanut butter, garlic, sugar substitute, and red pepper flakes. Divide among small individual serving bowls. Set aside.

To serve, soak the rice paper rounds in warm water to cover for about 1 minute, until softened. Drain on a kitchen towel and place on a plate or work surface. Place

½ lettuce leaf at the end of the wrapper closest to you. Top with ⅛ of the vegetables. Roll the wrapper over tightly once, then turn in the ends. Continue to roll the wrapper and filling over onto itself to make a spring roll. Serve at once, either whole or cut in half, with dipping sauce on the side.

Makes 8 large rolls.

JOSLIN CHOICES (1 roll): 2 carbohydrate (bread/starch)
PER SERVING: 140 calories (10% calories from fat), 2 g total fat (0 saturated fat), 5 g protein,
    27 g carbohydrates, 2 g dietary fiber, 3 mg cholesterol, 261 mg sodium, 153 mg potassium

Eggplant Terrine with Basil Tomato Sauce

Roasting eggplant leaves the flesh soft and sweet, making it wonderful for timbales, soufflés, and this terrine. Frequently paired with tomatoes and fresh basil, eggplant prepared in this manner is a festive appetizer or can be a light main course, needing only a green salad and crusty whole wheat bread to complete the meal.

The juice from the pressed cooked eggplant gives the sauce a subtle flavor that will delight you and your guests.

> *olive oil cooking spray*
> *4 small eggplants (about 4 pounds total)*
> *½ cup bread crumbs*
> *¼ cup grated Parmesan cheese*
> *6 tablespoons egg substitute*
> *3 large egg whites*
> *⅛ teaspoon salt (optional)*
> *freshly ground pepper to taste*
>
> BASIL TOMATO SAUCE
> *¾ cup juice from eggplants*
> *1 14½-ounce can no-salt-added diced tomatoes, well drained*
> *3 tablespoons chopped fresh basil*
> *extra basil sprigs for garnish (optional)*

Preheat the oven to 450°F. Lightly coat a nonstick baking sheet with cooking spray.

Cut the tops off 3 eggplants and cut in half lengthwise. Score the flesh slightly. Place the 6 halves on the prepared baking sheet. Bake until the eggplants are very soft and caramelized, about 40 minutes. Remove from the oven and, when cool enough to handle, scoop out the flesh into a strainer that is suspended over a bowl. Using the back of a large spoon, press the eggplant flesh to extract its juices. Let the eggplant drain for 10 minutes, then press again with the back of a spoon. Repeat this procedure twice. Place the juice in a small saucepan to make the sauce. There should be ¾ to 1 cup juice.

Slice the remaining eggplant lengthwise into 8 thin slices. Spray both sides with cooking spray and bake until soft, about 10 to 15 minutes. Set aside.

In a bowl, combine the drained eggplant, bread crumbs, Parmesan cheese, and egg substitute. In a mixing bowl, beat the egg whites until they form stiff peaks. Carefully fold into the eggplant mixture. Season with salt (if using) and pepper.

Lightly coat a nonstick 8½ x 4-inch loaf pan with cooking spray and line the bottom with 2 slices of the baked eggplant. Place the remaining slices vertically around the inside of the loaf pan, allowing the ends to hang over the sides of the pan. Fill the center with the eggplant mixture. Fold the overhanging slices of eggplant over the top. Bake for 30 minutes. Turn out onto a cutting board or serving platter.

To make the sauce, combine the reserved juices from the cooked, pressed eggplant with the diced tomatoes in a small saucepan. Add the basil and simmer over medium heat for 5 minutes.

To serve, place a slice of terrine on a small plate and surround with 2 tablespoons of sauce. Garnish with fresh basil sprigs, if using.

Makes 8 appetizer or 4 main course servings.

JOSLIN CHOICES (appetizer): ½ very-low-fat protein, I carbohydrate (bread/starch)
PER SERVING: 131 calories (15% calories from fat), 2 g total fat (I g saturated fat), 7 g
    protein, 23 g carbohydrates, 6 g dietary fiber, 3 mg cholesterol, 206 mg sodium, 759 mg
    potassium
JOSLIN CHOICES (main course): I low-fat protein, 2 carbohydrate (bread/starch)
PER SERVING: 261 calories (15% calories from fat), 5 g total fat (2 g saturated fat), 15 g
    protein, 45 g carbohydrates, 13 g dietary fiber, 5 mg cholesterol, 412 mg sodium, 1,518 mg
    potassium

Vegetable Strudel

*P*ackaged filo dough takes the mystery and hard work out of making a strudel. Just follow the directions on the package for thawing, and handle the sheets of dough gently so they remain intact. The variety of vegetables and herbs that can be used in a strudel depends only on what's freshest at the market. The end result will be crisp vegetables in a buttery-tasting crust. This is one of our favorite combinations—an easy-to-make appetizer or, when cut into quarters, main course.

olive oil cooking spray
½ small red onion, thinly sliced
1 medium red bell pepper, cored, deveined, and thinly sliced
1 medium yellow bell pepper, cored, deveined, and thinly sliced
2 small zucchini (10 ounces total), thinly sliced
1 4-ounce portobello mushroom, halved and thinly sliced
⅓ cup fresh basil, cut into thin strips
freshly ground pepper to taste
¼ teaspoon kosher salt (optional)
6 sheets filo dough (about 18 x 14 inches each), thawed if frozen
butter-flavored cooking spray
10 baby spinach leaves, stems removed, washed, and dried
¼ cup grated skim milk cheddar cheese
½ teaspoon sesame seeds

Preheat the oven to 425°F. Lightly coat a large skillet with cooking spray and place over medium-high heat.

Add the onion, bell peppers, zucchini, and mushroom. Cook, stirring occasionally, until the vegetables are soft, about 8 minutes. Stir in the basil, pepper, and salt (if using). Set aside to cool.

Lay a sheet of filo on a work surface and lightly coat with butter-flavored spray; top with a second sheet. Continue until you have 6 layers, lightly spraying each sheet.

Place the spinach along one short edge of the filo, leaving about 1½ inches empty around the spinach on each side and the bottom. Sprinkle grated cheese over the spinach. Top with the cooled vegetables. Fold the short edge over the vegetables and fold in the long edges. Roll the filo and filling over onto itself to form a strudel roll. Place seam side down on a nonstick baking pan.

Spray the strudel with butter spray and sprinkle with sesame seeds. Bake until golden brown, about 25 minutes. Serve warm.

Makes 8 appetizer or 4 main course servings.

JOSLIN CHOICES (appetizer): 2 vegetables
PER SERVING: 71 calories (17% calories from fat), 1 g total fat (0 saturated fat), 4 g protein,
    12 g carbohydrates, 2 g dietary fiber, 1 mg cholesterol, 158 mg sodium, 297 mg potassium
JOSLIN CHOICES (main course): 1 carbohydrate (1 bread/starch), 1 vegetable (½ fat)
PER SERVING: 143 calories (17% calories from fat), 3 g total fat (1 g saturated fat), 8 g protein,
    24 g carbohydrates, 4 g dietary fiber, 1 mg cholesterol, 315 mg sodium, 594 mg potassium

Gourmet Popped Corn

*P*opcorn may be America's favorite snack food, and when popped without oil or butter it's 27 calories per cup. Since it's a whole grain with a high fiber content, it has a well-deserved recommendation as a high-fiber snack.

And more than all of that, popcorn is just fun to eat. Combined with a few staples from your kitchen pantry, it'll transform into a snack to satisfy the kid in you for just pennies.

Here are three of our favorite ways to prepare it.

Bayou Blast

1 quart hot air–popped corn
butter-flavored cooking spray or butter-flavored granules, reconstituted
½ teaspoon paprika
½ teaspoon salt (optional)
¼ teaspoon cayenne pepper
¼ teaspoon onion powder
⅛ teaspoon crushed dried oregano
⅛ teaspoon crushed dried thyme
⅛ teaspoon freshly ground black pepper

Put the popcorn in a clean large paper grocery bag. Lightly coat the popcorn with cooking spray. In a small bowl, combine the paprika, salt (if using), cayenne pepper, onion powder, oregano, thyme, and black pepper. Sprinkle over the popcorn. Close the bag and shake several times to evenly coat the popcorn. Pour into a bowl and serve warm.

Makes 1 serving.

JOSLIN CHOICES: 1½ carbohydrate (bread/starch)

PER SERVING: 131 calories (11% calories from fat), 2 g fat (0 saturated fat), 4 g protein, 27 g carbohydrates, 5 g dietary fiber, 0 cholesterol, 943 mg sodium, 145 mg potassium

Chocolate

1 quart hot air–popped corn
butter-flavored cooking spray or butter-flavored granules, reconstituted
3 tablespoons powdered cocoa mix presweetened with sugar substitute
1 teaspoon ground cinnamon

Put the popcorn in a clean large paper grocery bag. Lightly coat the popcorn with cooking spray. Add the cocoa mix and cinnamon. Close the bag and shake several times to evenly coat the popcorn. Pour into a bowl and serve warm.

Makes 1 serving.

JOSLIN CHOICES: 1½ carbohydrate (bread/starch)

PER SERVING: 140 calories (9% calories from fat), 2 g fat (0 saturated fat), 5 g protein, 29 g carbohydrates, 6 g dietary fiber, 0 cholesterol, 45 mg sodium, 209 mg potassium

Dilled Ranch*

1 quart hot air–popped corn
butter-flavored cooking spray or butter-flavored granules, reconstituted
2 tablespoons dried ranch-style dip mix
1 teaspoon dried dill weed

*Recipe not recommended for a low-sodium diet.

1 teaspoon finely grated lemon zest
½ teaspoon onion powder

Put the popcorn in a clean large paper grocery bag. Lightly coat the popcorn with cooking spray. In a small bowl, combine the dip mix, dill weed, lemon zest, and onion powder. Sprinkle over the popcorn. Close the bag and shake several times to evenly coat the popcorn. Pour into a bowl and serve warm.

Makes 1 serving.

JOSLIN CHOICES: 2½ carbohydrate (2½ bread/starch)
PER SERVING: 200 calories (7% calories from fat), 1 g fat (0 saturated fat), 4 g protein, 41 g
    carbohydrate, 5 g dietary fiber, 0 cholesterol, 1,989 mg sodium, 286 mg potassium

Mixed Berry Yogurt Smoothie

*N*eed a quick breakfast for the family or a pick-me-up when the low-sugar blues hit in the afternoon? This recipe for a smoothie fits the bill. Try adding your favorite juices or frozen fruit and garnish with any fresh fruit or mint.

1 16-ounce container plain nonfat yogurt
1 12-ounce package no-sugar-added frozen mixed berries
1 packet sugar substitute
¼ teaspoon pure vanilla extract
½ cup ice cubes
½ cup fresh orange juice
strawberry slices and mint sprigs for garnish

In a blender or food processor fitted with a metal blade, place the yogurt, frozen berries, sugar substitute, and vanilla. Process until the mixture becomes smooth. Add the ice cubes and juice. Process again until all the ice cubes have been incorporated.

Pour into 4 glasses and garnish with slices of strawberry and a sprig of mint.

Makes 4 servings.

JOSLIN CHOICES: 1½ carbohydrate (1 fruit, ½ nonfat milk)

PER SERVING: 103 calories (3% calories from fat), 0 total fat (0 saturated fat), 6 g protein,
23 g carbohydrates, 2 g dietary fiber, 2 mg cholesterol, 69 mg sodium, 148 mg potassium

---

Smoothies

Smoothies are the rage everywhere—you can enjoy them at stands in most shopping malls, and there are even a couple of cookbooks devoted to the subject. Be wary of smoothies away from home, as they may be loaded with carbs and fat.

Smoothies are so easy to make, all you really need is a blender or food processor and a few simple ingredients. Keep the blender handy on the counter for making early-morning breakfast smoothies and midafternoon pick-me-ups.

Here's the basic recipe; add your choice within each of the four parts in the order given:

The Base: skim milk, fresh fruit juice, nonfat yogurt, or nonfat frozen yogurt

Fruit: fresh, frozen, or canned with no sugar added

Some Flavorings: vanilla extract, ground nutmeg, ground cinnamon, coffee, or unsweetened chocolate

Sweeteners: sugar, sugar substitutes, honey, sugar-free maple syrup, or all-fruit spreads (add the sweetener last; many fruits, such as ripe banana, will already be sweet enough)

Now blend to desired consistency and serve. Use the Joslin Choices (page 233) to figure out your carbs.

SALADS AND SALAD DRESSINGS

A Primer on Lettuce and Greens

The darker the lettuce or greens in your salad bowl, the better. With the wonderful array now available to us, long gone is the day when salad meant iceberg lettuce. Your mom and Popeye were right about eating spinach—just 1 cup of raw spinach (or chard, collards, mustards, watercress, or dandelions) provides 100 percent of the USDA requirement for vitamin A, with only 7 calories.

Here are your choices:

Arugula: dark green with a peppery taste; small leaves are the mildest

Belgian endive: white, yellow-edged crunchy leaves with a slightly bitter bite

Bibb lettuce: small head with pale to medium green tender leaves with a sweet, subtle taste

Boston lettuce: loose head with pale green leaves and a buttery flavor

Cabbage, Chinese: most delicately flavored of all cabbages, with very light green, crinkly leaves in an elongated head

Cabbage, green: pale green, crisp leaves with a bite

Cabbage, red: crisp purple leaves with a bite

Chicory (curly endive): curly and crisp green leaves with a pale center

Dandelion: pale young leaves are best

Escarole: crisp light-green leaves with a pale heart

Frisée: sweetest of the chicory family, with pale green to almost white curly, mildly bitter leaves

Iceberg: crisp, cool leaves with very mild flavor

Kale: dark red or green robust-flavored leaves

Loose-leaf lettuce: young, soft, red or green leaves with sweet flavor

Mâche (lamb's lettuce, corn salad, or field salad): small green leaves with sweet-nutty flavor

Mesclun: mixture of very young tender greens, herbs, and sometimes edible flowers (see page 49)

Radicchio: brilliant, ruby-colored leaves in a cabbage-like head with slightly bitter, peppery taste

Romaine: long, crisp, succulent, medium green or red leaves with a fresh, sweet flavor

Spinach: long, pear-shaped smooth leaves with a spicy flavor

Watercress: tiny, round, glossy dark green leaves with a spicy, peppery taste

Belgian Endive and Watercress Salad with Blue Cheese Toasts

*B*elgian endive is a small cylindrical head of tightly packed leaves. To retain its creamy color, it is grown in the dark. Buy crisp, firm heads with only a bit of green at the tips. Keep them refrigerated, wrapped in a paper towel in a plastic bag, for no more than one day.

BLUE CHEESE TOASTS
8¼-inch-thick slices French baguette, about 2 inches in diameter
olive oil cooking spray
4 teaspoons crumbled blue cheese

VINAIGRETTE
1½ tablespoons raspberry vinegar
⅛ teaspoon salt (optional)
1 scallion, white part only, minced
1½ tablespoons olive oil
freshly ground pepper to taste

SALAD
½ pound watercress, thick stems discarded
¾ pound white Belgian endive
1 large ripe red Comice pear (about 8 ounces), quartered and cored

Preheat the broiler.

To make the toasts, place the thin rounds of French bread on a baking sheet and lightly coat with cooking spray. Spread ½ teaspoon blue cheese on each slice and broil until bubbling and browned. Watch carefully; once it begins to brown, it will finish quickly. Remove and set aside.

Prepare the vinaigrette by whisking the vinegar and salt (if using) in a small cup. Mix in the scallion, olive oil, and pepper. Set aside.

In a salad bowl, place the watercress, separated into short leafy pieces. Just before serving, cut the endives in half lengthwise, removing and discarding the core. Cut the endives into ¼-inch-thick slices.

To serve, toss the greens with the vinaigrette and divide among 4 salad plates. Cut each quarter of pear into 3 thin slices and fan on top of the greens. Top with 2 blue cheese toasts.

Makes 4 servings.

JOSLIN CHOICES: 1½ carbohydrate (1 bread/starch, ½ fruit), 2 fat
PER SERVING: 229 calories (34% calories from fat), 9 g total fat (2 g saturated fat), 6 g
    protein, 33 g carbohydrates, 8 g dietary fiber, 2 mg cholesterol, 312 mg sodium, 338 mg
    potassium

Green Salad with Herbs and Warm Goat Cheese

*Y*ears ago we took a cooking class from Patricia Wells. She prepared a salad redolent of fresh herbs, as they do in Provence, where herbs grow wild everywhere. This simple bistro salad has now become popular in trendy restaurants across the country. If your market sells a fresh mesclun mix, all the better, but packaged baby greens will also make a nifty salad.

> *8 cups mesclun or mixed baby greens, rinsed and dried*
> *1 tablespoon fresh thyme leaves*
> *1 tablespoon minced fresh basil*
> *1 tablespoon minced fresh dill*
> *1 tablespoon minced fresh oregano*
> *1 tablespoon minced flat-leaf parsley*
> *4 ounces low-fat goat cheese, cut into 6 rounds*
> *Basic Oil and Vinegar Vinaigrette (page 69)*

salt to taste (optional)
freshly ground pepper to taste

Place the mesclun and herbs in a large salad bowl. Set aside.

Preheat the oven to 400°F. Line a small baking sheet with parchment. Arrange the goat cheese rounds on parchment paper. Place in the oven and warm until the cheese begins to melt, about 2 minutes.

To serve, drizzle the vinaigrette over the greens and herbs. Season with salt (if using) and pepper and toss to evenly coat the greens. Divide the greens among 6 plates and place a warmed goat cheese round at the edge of each plate. Serve at once.

Makes 6 servings.

JOSLIN CHOICES (with dressing): 1 medium-fat protein, 1 fat
PER SERVING: 125 calories (73% calories from fat), 10 g total fat (5 g saturated fat), 5 g
    protein, 3 g carbohydrates, 1 g dietary fiber, 15 mg cholesterol, 117 mg sodium, 281 mg
    potassium

Hearts of Romaine with Basil-Yogurt Dressing

*T*his is an interesting combination of flavors and a welcome change from the traditional iceberg lettuce salad.

1 large head romaine lettuce

DRESSING
½ cup loosely packed fresh basil leaves
¾ cup plain nonfat yogurt
1 teaspoon Dijon mustard
1 teaspoon minced shallots
1 teaspoon fresh lemon juice
½ teaspoon grated lemon zest
¼ teaspoon freshly ground pepper
2 tablespoons chopped walnuts for garnish

Remove the dark green outer leaves from the romaine and discard or reserve for another use. Tear the remaining leaves into bite-size pieces (you should get about 6 cups). Rinse the lettuce and spin dry, or wrap in paper towels and refrigerate until ready to use.

To make the dressing, in a food processor fitted with a metal blade, process the basil, yogurt, mustard, shallots, lemon juice, lemon zest, and pepper until smooth. Transfer the mixture to a covered container and refrigerate until ready to use. (Makes about ¾ cup.)

To assemble the salad, divide the lettuce among 6 chilled salad plates. Top each salad with 2 tablespoons of the dressing and sprinkle each with 1 teaspoon chopped walnuts. Serve at once.

Makes 6 servings.

JOSLIN CHOICES: 1 vegetable
PER SERVING: 66 calories (24% calories from fat), 2 g total fat (0 saturated fat), 5 g protein,
    9 g carbohydrates, 5 g dietary fiber, 1 mg cholesterol, 48 mg sodium, 23 mg potassium
JOSLIN CHOICES (dressing only): 1 vegetable
PER SERVING: 40 calories (6% calories from fat), 0 total fat (0 saturated fat), 3 g protein, 7 g
    carbohydrates, 3 g dietary fiber, 1 mg cholesterol, 42 mg sodium, 6 mg potassium

Making Your Own Mesclun

Right next to the expensive mesclun mix, you're likely to find bunches of fresh arugula, mâche, and baby spinach; small heads of radicchio and frisée. To a mixture of these, you can add a handful of whole fresh basil leaves, cilantro, parsley, chives, sorrel, and mint for additional flavor, creating your own personal blend of mesclun. Since tender baby greens are highly perishable, look for leaves that are brightly colored, light and fluffy, and fresh scented. Rinse and spin them dry or air-dry on paper towels as soon as you get home. The mesclun will keep for a couple of days in an aerated plastic bag in the refrigerator.

Apple and Jicama Salad

*I*f you haven't tried jicama, look for this brown-skinned root vegetable in your market near the chiles and exotic produce. Once you taste its sweet, crunchy flesh, you'll love it and serve it often. The trick with jicama is not to peel it until you're ready to use it. Unpeeled and refrigerated, it will last up to five days.

The contrast of tart apple and sweet jicama combined with Tex-Mex spices makes this salad perfect for a south-of-the-border dinner.

1 medium jicama (about 10 ounces), peeled
1 large Granny Smith apple

VINAIGRETTE
juice of 1 lime
1 small clove garlic, minced
½ teaspoon ground cumin
¼ teaspoon Dijon mustard
1½ tablespoons olive oil
1½ tablespoons chopped fresh mint

4 leaves red leaf lettuce
1 tablespoon dry-roasted sesame seeds
extra mint for garnish

Slice the jicama into thin rounds and then cut into narrow strips. Place in a bowl. Quarter the apple and core. Do not peel. Cut into thin slices. Add to the bowl.

To prepare the vinaigrette, in a small cup, combine the lime juice, garlic, cumin, mustard, oil, and chopped mint; mix well. Pour over the jicama and apples. Toss and set aside until ready to serve.

To serve, place a lettuce leaf on each salad plate. Top with one-quarter of the jicama salad and sprinkle each with a bit of sesame seeds. Garnish with extra mint.

Makes 4 servings.

JOSLIN CHOICES: 1 vegetable, 1 fat

PER SERVING: 108 calories (50% calories from fat), 6 g total fat (1 g saturated fat), 2 g protein, 13 g carbohydrates, 5 g dietary fiber, 0 cholesterol, 13 mg sodium, 202 mg potassium

Mixed Citrus Salad

*T*his bright salad had been a favorite of ours for years, especially when we grew our own citrus while living in southern California. Happily, we get excellent citrus where we now live, especially the ruby red grapefruit of south Texas. On a cold, wet day its sweetness is particularly pleasing.

For the mixed greens, we usually pick an organic mix of mesclun—a blend of 8 to 12 different types of baby lettuce leaves, wild greens, savory herbs, and edible flower petals that our supermarket carries in the produce section. If your market doesn't have blood oranges, substitute a Mineola or Mandarin orange.

> *1 large navel orange*
> *1 lemon*
> *boiling water*
> *1 blood orange*
> *1 large ruby red grapefruit*
> *1 lime*
> *2 honey tangerines*
> *1 tablespoon sugar*
> *1 tablespoon sherry vinegar*
> *1 tablespoon canola oil*
> *6 cups mesclun or mixed baby greens, rinsed and crisped*
> *2 large shallots, minced*
> *3 tablespoons minced fresh basil*
> *1 tablespoon chopped walnuts*
> *freshly ground pepper to taste*

Using a citrus zester or a handheld fine grater, zest the navel orange and lemon. Place the zest in a small bowl and cover with boiling water. Let stand for 3 minutes; drain and scatter the zest strips on paper towels to dry. Set aside.

Working over a large bowl to catch any juice, peel the orange, lemon, blood orange, grapefruit, lime, and tangerines, removing all the white pith. Thinly slice each fruit crosswise and discard any seeds. Set the fruit slices aside.

To the collected fruit juices, whisk in the sugar, vinegar, and oil. Set aside.

To arrange the salads, divide the mesclun among 6 large plates. Arrange the citrus slices on top in a decorative pattern, mixing the colors, sizes, and flavors. In a small bowl, combine the shallots, basil, and walnuts; sprinkle the mixture over each salad. Again whisk the dressing and drizzle over each salad. Grind pepper on top and sprinkle with the reserved citrus zests. Serve at once.

Makes 6 servings.

JOSLIN CHOICES: 1 carbohydrate (fruit), ½ fat
PER SERVING: 119 calories (23% calories from fat), 3 g total fat (0 saturated fat), 2 g protein,
    23 g carbohydrates, 5 g dietary fiber, 0 cholesterol, 18 mg sodium, 502 mg potassium

Southwestern Corn and Peach Salad

*W*hen summer corn is freshly picked and delivered daily (sometimes twice daily) to your market, you'll find this vibrant summer salad perfect for a buffet or a meal of different salads. We add chicken or vegetable broth to the corn cooking liquid to infuse the salad with a rich sweetness.

3 cups water
1 cup canned low-fat, low-sodium chicken or vegetable broth
4 medium ears fresh corn, shucked and kernels cut from cobs
1 medium roasted red bell pepper packed in brine, drained and coarsely chopped
1 small white onion, chopped
4 ounces jicama, peeled and cut into thin julienne strips
2 tablespoons olive oil
2 tablespoons fresh lime juice
1 red or green jalapeño chile pepper, seeded and minced
¼ teaspoon cumin seed
1 small head radicchio, separated into leaves

2 large ripe peaches
¼ cup minced mixed fresh herbs: cilantro, chervil, basil, mint, or flat-leaf parsley

In a medium saucepan, bring the water and broth to a rapid boil. Add the corn and blanch for 2 minutes. Drain and refresh under running cold water. Drain again. Place in a large bowl; add the roasted bell pepper, onion, and jicama.

In a measuring cup, whisk together the olive oil, lime juice, jalapeño, and cumin seed. Pour over the corn mixture and toss. (The salad can be made ahead up to this point, covered, and refrigerated.)

When ready to serve, arrange the radicchio leaves on a large platter. Wash and peel the peaches (if necessary, dip them in boiling water for 1 minute to facilitate removing the skin). Cut in half and remove and discard the pits. Slice the peaches into wedges and add to the corn mixture. Toss and spoon into the radicchio leaves. Sprinkle with the herbs and serve.

Makes 6 servings.

JOSLIN CHOICES: I carbohydrate (bread/starch), I fat
PER SERVING: 133 calories (35% calories from fat), 6 g total fat (I g saturated fat), 3 g
    protein, 20 g carbohydrates, 4 g dietary fiber, I mg cholesterol, 31 mg sodium, 343 mg
    potassium

Citrus Zest

*I*n this book we call for a lot of zest, the perfumey outermost skin layer of citrus fruit, to take advantage of the intense aroma and flavor of citrus in the peel of lemons and oranges. Zest adds an amazing flavor to everything from soup to dessert.

You can buy a citrus zester in gourmet cookware shops and many supermarkets. It makes it easy to remove the zest from the bitter white pith underneath. You can also use a handheld grater to remove the zest; just be careful not to nick your knuckles. Once the zest is removed, mince it finely unless otherwise directed by the recipe.

Chopping Fresh Herbs

Chopping fresh herbs can be difficult if the leaves are still damp. The chopping brings out extra moisture and the leaves will clump together as you chop. Always rinse the leaves and let them completely air-dry on paper towels before starting the chopping process; they'll be easier to chop. If you're not adept with a knife, put the tender herbs into a glass measuring cup, and with kitchen shears held straight down into the cup, you can easily and rapidly snip the herbs by merely opening and closing the shears.

Peach and Sweet Onion Salad

This recipe was recently served at a summer Texas barbecue—the peaches, perfectly ripe and juicy, were a delicious contrast to the crunchy sweet onion, lightly dressed with lemon juice and a "kick" of hot pepper sauce. Served over a mixture of baby salad greens with a generous portion of arugula, they make a stunning salad for summer picnics and cookouts.

6 ripe peaches (about 1½ pounds total), peeled and thinly sliced
1 medium sweet onion (such as Texas 1015, Vidalia, Walla Walla, or Maui), peeled, halved lengthwise, and cut into thin crosswise slices
¼ cup fresh lemon juice
¼ teaspoon hot pepper sauce, or to taste
¼ teaspoon kosher salt (optional)
freshly ground pepper to taste
6 cups mixed baby salad greens, rinsed and crisped
2 cups fresh arugula, tough stems removed, rinsed and crisped

In a large bowl, combine the peach and onion slices. In a small cup, whisk together the lemon juice, hot pepper sauce, salt (if using), and pepper. Pour over the peach mixture and toss lightly to coat evenly. Set aside for at least 30 minutes to allow the flavors to combine.

When ready to serve, combine the baby greens and arugula. Divide among 6 salad plates and top each portion with the peach and onion slices. Drizzle with some of the juices from the bowl and serve at once.

Makes 6 servings.

JOSLIN CHOICES: 1 carbohydrate (fruit)

PER SERVING: 66 calories (4% calories from fat), 0 total fat (0 saturated fat), 2 g protein, 16 g carbohydrates, 4 g dietary fiber, 0 cholesterol, 17 mg sodium, 449 mg potassium

Tomato and Mango Salad on Arugula and Curly Endive

*W*hen summer's bounty of luscious tomatoes is available, try this delightful combination. At other times, substitute ripe plum tomatoes or hothouse tomatoes if affordable.

> *3 medium tomatoes (about ¾ pound total)*
> *1 large ripe mango*
> *1 scallion, white part and 1 inch green, chopped*
> *3 tablespoons chopped fresh basil*

> VINAIGRETTE
> *1½ tablespoons white wine vinegar*
> *1½ tablespoons olive oil*
> *⅛ teaspoon salt (optional)*
> *freshly ground pepper to taste*

> *2½ ounces arugula, rinsed and dried*
> *¼ pound curly endive, rinsed, dried, and torn into bite-size pieces*
> *extra basil for garnish*

Quarter the tomatoes, then cut into ½-inch-thick crosswise slices. Place in a bowl. Peel the mango and cut into 1-inch dice. Add to the bowl along with the scallion and basil. Stir to combine.

To prepare the vinaigrette, in a cup, whisk the vinegar, olive oil, salt (if using), and pepper. Drizzle over the tomato-mango mixture and set aside until ready to serve.

Combine the arugula and endive. Divide among 4 salad plates. Top each with the tomato-mango combination. Garnish with basil.

Makes 4 servings.

JOSLIN CHOICES: 1 carbohydrate (fruit), 1 fat

PER SERVING: 107 calories (43% calories from fat), 6 g total fat (1 g saturated fat), 2 g protein, 15 g carbohydrates, 3 g dietary fiber, 0 cholesterol, 80 mg sodium, 443 mg potassium

How to Handle a Mango

Although we have called for fresh mangos in our two previous cookbooks, when we teach cooking classes or do book signings, we're frequently asked how to free the mango fruit from its large pit without turning the whole fruit into a mushy mess.

Anyone can master a mango. First, pick a mango that has a sweet, floral scent. It should be firm but give slightly to the touch—much like a peach or nectarine does when it's ripe; avoid any soft or bruised mangoes.

Hold the mango in the palm of one hand with its narrower profile facing you. Using a small, sharp knife or sturdy vegetable peeler, peel the skin away from the flesh. After determining the location of the ½- to ¾-inch-thick pit (it runs the length of the fruit between the two fleshier sides), slowly cut through the mango lengthwise down the side of the pit until the fleshy side is cut off. Repeat on the other side. Cut the remaining fruit from the pit. Then cut the fruit into thin slices or dice, according to the recipe directions. If desired, scrape any remaining flesh from the mango pit and add to the fruit.

Watermelon Salad

*T*his lively salad needs to be assembled just before serving. If made too far in advance, the watermelon releases its juice and makes the mixture watery. Since we can now buy excellent watermelon year-round, this is a favorite refreshing salad to accompany a spicy meal. You may substitute shredded part-skim mozzarella for the low-fat feta cheese for an equally delicious flavor.

> *6 cups diced cold seedless watermelon*
> *1 cup diced hothouse (seedless) cucumber*
> *⅓ cup finely diced red onion*
> *1 cup coarsely chopped fresh mint*
> *¼ cup crumbled low-fat feta cheese*
> *¼ cup fresh lime juice*
> *additional mint leaves for garnish*

On a large platter, arrange the watermelon pieces. Scatter the cucumber, onion, and mint over the watermelon. Sprinkle with the feta cheese and drizzle with lime juice. Serve at once garnished with mint leaves.

Makes 6 servings.

JOSLIN CHOICES: 1 carbohydrate (fruit)
PER SERVING: 74 calories (17% calories from fat), 2 g total fat (1 g saturated fat), 3 g protein,
    14 g carbohydrates, 1 g dietary fiber, 3 mg cholesterol, 28 mg sodium, 223 mg potassium

Italian Roasted Beet Salad

*T*he combination of roasted beets, onions, and asparagus is well known and loved in Italy. To avoid turning your fingers pink, peel the beets before you bake them and slice the cooked beets directly into the bowl using a sharp fork to hold them steady.

> *1 pound small beets, peeled*
> *1 small onion, thinly sliced and separated into rings*

½ pound thin asparagus, woody ends discarded
olive oil cooking spray
1½ tablespoons olive oil
1 tablespoon balsamic vinegar
⅛ teaspoon sugar substitute
⅛ teaspoon kosher salt (optional)
freshly ground pepper to taste
4 cups torn romaine lettuce leaves

Preheat the oven to 350°F.

Place the peeled beets in aluminum foil and seal tightly. Bake for 45 minutes to an hour, until tender when pierced with a fork. Place in a bowl to cool. Raise the oven temperature to 400°F.

Place the onion rings and asparagus on a baking sheet and coat with cooking spray. Bake until the onion has begun to caramelize and the asparagus is browned, about 25 minutes, turning every 5 to 8 minutes. Remove from the oven and reserve the onion. Thinly slice the beets. Add the asparagus. Toss with the oil, vinegar, sugar substitute, salt (if using), and pepper.

To serve, divide the lettuce among 4 plates and top with the beet mixture. Garnish with some of the caramelized onions.

Makes 4 servings.

JOSLIN CHOICES: 2 vegetable, 1 fat
PER SERVING: 124 calories (37% calories from fat), 6 g total fat (1 g saturated fat), 4 g protein,
   17 g carbohydrates, 6 g dietary fiber, 0 cholesterol, 154 mg sodium, 715 mg potassium

Farmer's Market Corn and Tomato Salad

We're both fortunate to live in areas where farmers set up stalls in the heart of town to display rows of summer produce with high quality and low prices that make a drive from far away worthwhile. We come home with bags of fruits and vegetables, usually more than we really need, and invariably at least one bag holds vine-ripened tomatoes and corn still warm from the fields. This is one of our favorite ways to combine the two.

2 cups fresh corn kernels (cut from 4 large ears)
2 ripe tomatoes, seeded and coarsely chopped
4 scallions, white part and 1 inch green, chopped
2 tablespoons canola oil
2 tablespoons fresh lemon juice
1 tablespoon red wine vinegar
salt to taste (optional)
freshly ground pepper to taste

In a medium saucepan, blanch the corn kernels in boiling water to cover for 2 minutes. Drain.

In a medium bowl, toss the corn with the tomatoes and scallions. In a small bowl, whisk together the canola oil, lemon juice, and vinegar. Pour over the corn mixture and lightly toss. Season with salt (if using) and pepper. Toss again and serve at room temperature or chilled.

Makes 4 servings.

JOSLIN CHOICES: 1 carbohydrate (bread/starch), 1 fat
PER SERVING: 150 calories (44% calories from fat), 8 g total fat (1 g saturated fat), 3 g protein,
    20 g carbohydrates, 3 g dietary fiber, 0 cholesterol, 21 mg sodium, 437 mg potassium

Grilled Portobello Mushrooms over Spinach

*P*ortobellos are full-grown Italian cremini mushrooms that have wide, flat caps and very dark brown, almost black gills. Delicious grilled, they have a meaty texture and flavor. Here we've teamed portobellos with fresh spinach for an anytime salad, lightly dressed with a balsamic vinaigrette.

Be sure to try a grilled portobello on a bun with all of the fixings you used to put on hamburgers. The recipe's on page 95, and you'll be pleasantly surprised.

1 pound small spinach leaves
2 medium portobello mushrooms (about ¾ pound total)
olive oil cooking spray

VINAIGRETTE

1½ tablespoons balsamic vinegar
2 tablespoons olive oil
1 scallion, white part only, minced
1 clove garlic, minced
⅛ teaspoon salt (optional)
freshly ground pepper to taste

Preheat the broiler.

Wash the spinach well and remove any long thick stems. Dry and place in a salad bowl.

Lightly coat the mushrooms with cooking spray and broil about 4 inches from the source of heat for 5 minutes per side, turning once. Remove and slice into thin strips.

To prepare the vinaigrette, place the vinegar, oil, scallion, garlic, salt (if using), and pepper in a microwave-safe container. Cover and heat on high until the mixture is boiling, about 30 seconds.

Toss the hot dressing with the spinach. Divide among 4 salad plates and top with slices of warm mushroom. Serve immediately.

Makes 4 servings.

JOSLIN CHOICES: I vegetable, I fat
PER SERVING: I I 0 calories (51% calories from fat), 7 g total fat (I g saturated fat), 6 g
   protein, 9 g carbohydrates, 6 g dietary fiber, 0 cholesterol, 16 mg sodium, 64 mg potassium

Tunisian Potato, Cauliflower, and Chickpea Salad

*W*e've long been interested in the Tunisians' use of harissa, a fiery red pepper puree frequently sold in tubes and small jars in Middle Eastern shops. Here we've added harissa to a combination of potatoes, cauliflower, and chickpeas for a delicious year-round salad that's equally good warm or cold.

2 medium potatoes, scrubbed
1 small head cauliflower, broken into florets

1 15-ounce can chickpeas, rinsed and well drained

2 to 3 large cloves garlic

¼ cup fresh lemon juice

¼ teaspoon harissa (see below) or cayenne pepper

1 teaspoon ground cumin

1 teaspoon paprika

¾ cup plain low-fat yogurt

salt to taste (optional)

freshly ground pepper to taste

2 ounces low-fat feta cheese, crumbled

3 tablespoons chopped flat-leaf parsley or cilantro

In a large pot, cook the potatoes in boiling water to cover until almost tender, about 20 minutes. Add the cauliflower and continue to cook for another 5 minutes. Drain and refresh under cold water. Drain again. Slice the potatoes and place in a large bowl along with the cauliflower and drained chickpeas.

In a small bowl, combine the garlic, lemon juice, harissa, cumin, paprika, and yogurt. Spoon over the potato mixture and lightly toss to coat evenly. Taste and add salt (if using) and pepper. Serve warm or chilled, topped with the feta cheese and parsley.

Makes 6 servings.

JOSLIN CHOICES: 2 carbohydrate (bread/starch), 1 fat

PER SERVING: 195 calories (16% calories from fat), 4 g total fat (2 g saturated fat), 9 g protein,
34 g carbohydrates, 6 g dietary fiber, 11 mg cholesterol, 356 mg sodium, 594 mg potassium

Harissa

Once you've used this fiery red pepper sauce, you'll find lots of uses—add it to couscous and polenta or stir into nonfat yogurt to spoon over steamed vegetables or grated vegetable salads. Since it's very hot, use just a small amount in any one recipe. You can buy harissa in tubes or small jars in a Middle Eastern market, but it's quite easy to make your own, particularly if you grow your own hot chile peppers.

2 ounces small dried red chile peppers
4 cloves garlic, peeled and quartered
2 teaspoons caraway seed
1 teaspoon cumin seed
1 teaspoon coriander seed
½ teaspoon salt (optional)
7 tablespoons plus 1 teaspoon olive oil

In a small saucepan, bring the chiles and garlic to a boil in water to cover. Remove from the heat and let stand for 1 hour. Meanwhile, using a spice mill or a mortar and pestle, grind the spices. Set aside.

Remove the chiles and garlic, reserving the cooking liquid. Pat dry with paper towels and finely chop. Using the spice mill or mortar and pestle, grind or mash together the spices, chiles, and garlic until they form a thick paste. Stir in 7 tablespoons olive oil and 3 tablespoons of the reserved cooking liquid. Store in the refrigerator in a covered glass jar, covering the top of the paste with the remaining 1 teaspoon olive oil. Use within 3 months, replacing the top layer of olive oil after every use.

Makes about ¾ cup.

JOSLIN CHOICES: Free
PER ¼-TEASPOON SERVING: 8 calories (83% calories from fat), 1 g fat (0 saturated fat),
0 protein, 0 carbohydrates, 0 dietary fiber, 0 cholesterol, 8 mg sodium, 9 mg potassium

Root and Vegetable Slaw with Lemon Dressing

This fabulous tangy slaw is a perfect accompaniment to Portobello Mushroom Burgers (page 95) or Lentil Burgers (page 94). Although you can make the dressing earlier in the day, don't add it to the slaw until you're ready to serve, to ensure its crunchy texture and fresh flavor.

LEMON DRESSING

⅓ cup fat-free mayonnaise

⅓ cup fat-free sour cream

3 tablespoons fresh lemon juice

2 tablespoons olive oil

1 tablespoon white wine vinegar

1 tablespoon Dijon mustard

½ tablespoon prepared horseradish

1 teaspoon grated lemon zest

1 small clove garlic, minced

½ teaspoon salt (optional)

½ teaspoon celery seeds

½ teaspoon freshly ground pepper

SLAW

1 large knob celery root (about 1 pound), peeled

1 medium bulb fennel (about ½ pound), trimmed and washed

1 small head red cabbage (about ¾ pound), cored and tough outer leaves discarded

2 Belgian endives, core removed

In a bowl, whisk together the dressing ingredients. Transfer to a covered container and chill for at least 1 hour or up to 1 day.

Using a sharp knife or mandoline, cut the celery root, fennel, cabbage, and endive into thin slivers. Pour the dressing over the vegetables and toss. Serve at once.

Makes 8 servings.

JOSLIN CHOICES: 1 carbohydrate (bread/starch), 1 fat

PER SERVING: 115 calories (29% calories from fat), 4 g total fat (1 g saturated fat), 4 g
protein, 18 g carbohydrates, 5 g dietary fiber, 1 mg cholesterol, 368 mg sodium, 616 mg
potassium

Niçoise Salad

*I*n the south of France, this type of salad, served with a slice of crusty fresh country bread, makes memories at lunchtime. To serve for dinner, add white beans and perhaps some more vegetables, and you will think you are dining in Provence.

1 small head romaine lettuce (about 1 pound), rinsed and dried
½ pound cherry tomatoes, halved
½ pound fresh green beans, cooked and cut into 1½-inch pieces
½ pound small red potatoes, cooked and sliced
1 small cucumber, peeled, seeded, and thinly sliced
3 Niçoise or black ripe olives, pitted and chopped
1 hard-cooked egg white, chopped
3 tablespoons chopped fresh basil or flat-leaf parsley

VINAIGRETTE
2 tablespoons red wine vinegar
½ teaspoon Dijon mustard
¼ teaspoon anchovy paste (optional) or 2 teaspoons capers
1 tablespoon water
2½ tablespoons olive oil
freshly ground pepper to taste

Tear the romaine into bite-size pieces and place on a large platter. Arrange the tomatoes, green beans, potatoes, and cucumber on the lettuce in a decorative pattern. Sprinkle the top with olives, egg white, and basil.

To prepare the vinaigrette, in a small cup, mix together the vinegar, mustard, anchovy paste (if using), water, oil, and pepper. Drizzle over the salad and serve immediately.

Makes 4 servings.

JOSLIN CHOICES: 1 carbohydrate (bread/starch), 2 fat
PER SERVING: 193 calories (43% calories from fat), 10 g total fat (1 g saturated fat), 6 g protein, 24 g carbohydrates, 6 g dietary fiber, 0 cholesterol, 90 mg sodium, 964 mg potassium

Japanese Seaweed Salad

*T*he growing popularity of Japanese food in this country has produced a healthy addition to our eating experience. Even supermarkets now have sushi bars where you can watch a sushi chef prepare your meal. This type of salad is frequently served at sushi bars, and it's also terrific when mixed with rice. The typical seaweed used is arame, which comes dried. It is cut into long, thin strips after harvesting. Look for it in Asian markets or natural food stores.

¼ cup dried arame
1 1-pound English cucumber, peeled and very thinly sliced
2 radishes, very thinly sliced
⅛ teaspoon kosher salt (optional)
⅛ teaspoon sugar substitute
2 tablespoons rice wine vinegar
4 whole radishes, cut into flowers, for garnish

Rinse the arame in cold water, then soak in cold water for 5 minutes, drain, and place in a small saucepan. Cover the seaweed with fresh water. Simmer for 10 minutes. Drain, place in a salad bowl, and let cool.

Add the cucumber and sliced radishes to the arame, along with the salt (if using), sugar substitute, and vinegar. Mix well to combine.

To serve, divide among 4 Japanese rice bowls and garnish with radish flowers.

Makes 4 servings.

JOSLIN CHOICES: 1 vegetable
PER SERVING: 19 calories (9% calories from fat), 0 total fat (0 saturated fat), 1 g protein, 4 g
    carbohydrates, 1 g dietary fiber, 0 cholesterol, 68 mg sodium, 19 mg potassium

Spinach and Tempeh Salad with Wasabi Dressing

*W*hen you can't think of one more way to serve greens and you want some protein at the same time, remember this salad. Tempeh is made from cooked soybeans and needs to be steamed for 20 minutes before you use it. It is very absorbent, so it needs to be marinated for only about 15 minutes.

MARINADE
½ teaspoon wasabi powder
1 teaspoon water
1 teaspoon reduced-sodium soy sauce
¼ teaspoon sugar substitute
⅛ teaspoon dark sesame oil

WASABI DRESSING
1 teaspoon wasabi powder
1½ teaspoons water
1 tablespoon white wine vinegar
1 teaspoon reduced-sodium soy sauce
1 tablespoon canola oil
¼ teaspoon sugar substitute

4 ounces tempeh, steamed for 20 minutes, cooled, and crumbled
1 pound baby spinach leaves, washed and crisped
1 tablespoon toasted sesame seeds

To prepare the marinade, dissolve the wasabi in the water. Add the soy sauce, sugar substitute, and sesame oil.

To make the dressing, dissolve the wasabi in the water and whisk in the vinegar, soy sauce, oil, and sugar substitute.

Place the crumbled tempeh in a bowl. Pour the marinade over the tempeh and set aside for about 15 minutes.

Place the washed and dried spinach in a salad bowl. Drizzle the dressing over the spinach and toss well. Top with the tempeh and toss again. Sprinkle with the sesame seeds. Serve immediately.

Makes 4 servings.

JOSLIN CHOICES: I low-fat protein, I vegetable, I fat

PER SERVING: 128 calories (46% calories from fat), 6 g total fat (I g saturated fat), 8 g
   protein, 9 g carbohydrates, 2 g dietary fiber, 0 cholesterol, 93 mg sodium, 141 mg
   potassium

Italian Bread Salad

*T*his is a salad that we look forward to eating time after time when our gardens and farmer's markets are full of vine-ripened tomatoes and fresh basil. It's not a salad to be made with plastic-wrapped, overprocessed white bread, as the flavor relies heavily on using the right variety of bread. Look for an Italian bakery in your area and ask for a rustic whole-grain loaf that is coarsely textured and deeply flavored.

Fresh bread can ruin a bread salad. It becomes soggy too quickly. Be sure your bread is stale, ideally 3 days old. You can help fresh bread along by tearing it into chunks and drying it for about 30 minutes in a 375°F oven. Once that's done, the salad comes together quickly.

1 pound Italian country-style bread, about 3 days old, cut into 1-inch-thick slices
½ cup cold water
4 large tomatoes (about 1¾ pounds total), seeded and cut into chunks
1 large red onion, cut into ½-inch cubes
1 medium cucumber, peeled and cut into ½-inch cubes
½ cup loosely packed fresh basil leaves, torn into bite-size pieces

DRESSING
¼ cup red wine vinegar
1 large clove garlic, minced
3 tablespoons olive oil
2 tablespoons plain low-fat yogurt

Sprinkle the bread slices with water and let stand about 2 minutes. Gently squeeze the bread dry as you tear it into 1-inch cubes. Spread the bread pieces on paper towels and let air-dry for 20 minutes.

Meanwhile, combine the tomatoes, onion, cucumber, and basil in a large salad bowl. Add the dried bread cubes.

To prepare the dressing, in a small bowl, whisk together the vinegar, garlic, olive oil, and yogurt. Pour over the salad and toss to combine. Let stand until the bread has absorbed some of the dressing, about 20 minutes, and serve.

Makes 8 servings.

JOSLIN CHOICES: 2 carbohydrate (bread/starch), 1½ fat
PER SERVING: 235 calories (28% from fat), 8 g total fat (1 g saturated fat), 7 g protein, 36 g
  carbohydrates, 3 g dietary fiber, 0 cholesterol, 345 mg sodium, 387 mg potassium

Asian Vegetable Salad

*T*his refreshing salad is a welcome luncheon dish served with thin whole wheat pancakes or warmed tortillas for wrapping the salad. The rice wine vinegar and fresh ginger make the Asian flavors of the salad sing.

½ pound bean sprouts, roots pinched off
1 small carrot, julienned
2 ounces snow peas, strings removed and julienned
2½ ounces sliced water chestnuts (if using canned, rinse well and dry)
1½ tablespoons canola oil
1 scallion, white and 2 inches green, chopped
1 tablespoon rice vinegar
½ teaspoon grated fresh ginger
⅛ teaspoon kosher salt (optional)
freshly ground pepper to taste
1 tablespoon chopped fresh cilantro
1 tablespoon chopped dry-roasted peanuts

Blanch the bean sprouts in boiling water for 30 seconds. Using a slotted spoon, remove the sprouts and refresh in very cold water. Place in a large bowl.

Add the carrot and snow peas to the boiling water and blanch for 1 minute. Rinse under cold water and drain. Combine with the sprouts and water chestnuts.

Heat the oil in a nonstick pan and sauté the scallion over medium-high heat until wilted and lightly browned. Add the vinegar and ginger to the pan and remove from the heat. Pour over the vegetables and add salt (if using), pepper, and cilantro. Toss well and divide among 4 plates. Sprinkle with chopped peanuts.

Makes 4 servings.

JOSLIN CHOICES: I vegetable, I fat
PER SERVING: 100 calories (54% calories from fat), 6 g total fat (1 g saturated fat), 3 g
   protein, 9 g carbohydrates, 3 g dietary fiber, 0 cholesterol, 72 mg sodium, 19 mg potassium

Basic Oil and Vinegar Vinaigrette

1 shallot, minced
1 clove garlic, minced
1 tablespoon plus 1 teaspoon red wine vinegar
½ teaspoon cold water
2 tablespoons olive oil

In a small bowl, whisk the ingredients together. Set aside until ready to use, whisking again before adding to the salad.

Makes enough for 6 salads.

JOSLIN CHOICES (dressing only): I fat
PER SERVING: 42 calories (95% calories from fat), 5 g total fat (1 g saturated fat), 0 protein,
   0 carbohydrates, 0 dietary fiber, 0 cholesterol, I mg sodium, 8 mg potassium

VARIATIONS

Dijon Mustard: Add 1 teaspoon Dijon mustard.

Walnut Oil: Replace the red wine vinegar with white wine vinegar, and olive oil with walnut oil.

Balsamic Vinegar: Replace 1 teaspoon of the red wine vinegar with 1 teaspoon balsamic vinegar.

Creamy Tofu Salad Dressing

*W*hen you are in the mood for a thick and creamy salad dressing for your crisp greens, or you want a tasty dip for raw vegetables, this recipe is the answer.

7 ounces soft tofu, drained
2 tablespoons fat-free sour cream
2 tablespoons canola oil
3 tablespoons chopped flat-leaf parsley
3 tablespoons chopped fresh chives
1½ tablespoons chopped fresh tarragon leaves or ½ tablespoon crushed dried
1 clove garlic, peeled and cut into quarters

In a food processor fitted with a metal blade, place all the ingredients. Blend until the dressing is smooth and becomes a light shade of green. Refrigerate until ready to use.

Makes 1¼ cups.

JOSLIN CHOICES: 1 fat
PER ¼-CUP SERVING: 80 calories (73% calories from fat), 7 g total fat (1 g saturated fat), 3 g
    protein, 3 g carbohydrates, 0 dietary fiber, 0 cholesterol, 8 mg sodium, 114 mg potassium

Soups and Stews

Chilled Cucumber Soup

*T*his wonderfully refreshing summer soup has its origins in simple, humble ingredients—cucumber, chicken or vegetable broth, and milk. Fresh dill gives it character, and tiny bits of tomato, a colorful finish. When the temperature's soaring, it's a soup that you'll serve again and again.

1 large cucumber (about 1 pound)
1¼ cups canned low-fat, low-sodium chicken or vegetable broth
½ cup skim milk
¼ cup fresh lemon juice
salt to taste (optional)
freshly ground pepper to taste
¾ cup chopped fresh dill
1 medium plum tomato, seeded and finely minced

Peel the cucumber and cut in half lengthwise. Using a spoon, scoop out and discard the seeds. Cut the cucumber into chunks and place in a food processor fitted with a metal blade. Add the broth, milk, and lemon juice. Process until smooth. Taste and add salt (if using) and pepper. Stir in the dill. Transfer to a covered container and chill for at least 2 hours or up to 1 day.

To serve, stir the soup thoroughly. Ladle or pour it into chilled soup bowls or soup mugs. Sprinkle with minced tomato and serve.

Makes 4 servings.

JOSLIN CHOICES: I vegetable.
PER SERVING: 38 calories (15% calories from fat), I g total fat (0 saturated fat), 3 g protein, 6 g carbohydrates, I g dietary fiber, 2 mg cholesterol, 53 mg sodium, 225 mg potassium

Peeling and Seeding Tomatoes

Working with one tomato at a time, cut an X through the stem end. Drop the tomato into a pot of boiling water for 30 seconds. Immediately transfer it to a bowl of ice water to stop the cooking. Slip off the skin. Discard the skin and use the tomato as directed.

If seeding the tomato, cut it in half. Holding it over a strainer that has been set over a bowl to catch any juice, scoop out the seeds with your thumb or forefinger, catching the seeds in the strainer and the juice in the bowl. Discard the seeds and use the tomato and any juice as directed.

Fruited Gazpacho

This refreshing combination of fruits and vegetables will dazzle your eyes and your palate.

2 medium tomatoes, peeled and seeded

1 medium cantaloupe (about ¾ pound), peeled and seeded

½ large honeydew melon (about ¾ pound), peeled and seeded

1 small cucumber, peeled and seeded

1 medium sweet onion, peeled

1 medium yellow bell pepper, seeded

1 medium red bell pepper, seeded

2 jalapeño chile peppers, seeded

1 large clove garlic, minced

¼ cup chopped fresh cilantro

2 teaspoons grated orange zest

1 teaspoon grated lemon zest

1½ cups fresh orange juice

3 tablespoons fresh lemon juice

salt to taste (optional)

freshly ground pepper to taste
2 kiwifruit for garnish
cilantro sprigs for garnish

Using a food processor fitted with a metal blade, or by hand, finely chop the tomatoes, cantaloupe, honeydew, cucumber, onion, bell peppers, and chile peppers. Transfer to a large bowl. Stir in the garlic, cilantro, orange zest, lemon zest, orange juice, lemon juice, salt (if using), and pepper. Cover and chill for at least 1 hour.

Peel the kiwifruit and cut each into 8 thin crosswise slices. Ladle the gazpacho into chilled soup bowls and garnish each serving with 2 slices of overlapping kiwi slices and a sprig of cilantro.

Makes 8 servings.

JOSLIN CHOICES: 1½ carbohydrate (fruit)
PER SERVING: 106 calories (4% calories from fat), 0 total fat (0 saturated fat), 3 g protein,
25 g carbohydrates, 3 g dietary fiber, 0 cholesterol, 68 mg sodium, 655 mg potassium

Cold Yogurt and Garden Vegetable Soup

*T*his is a lovely summer or early fall soup to serve when it's too hot to cook. Since the vegetables need to marinate and chill for several hours, prepare them early in the day.

You'll need to make the yogurt cheese the night before, so plan ahead. Read the label of the yogurt and make sure there's no gelatin added.

YOGURT CHEESE
1 32-ounce container plain low-fat yogurt

SOUP
3 cups water
2 tablespoons white wine vinegar
1 medium onion, diced

1 clove garlic, minced
8 tiny new white potatoes (each about 1½ inches in diameter), scrubbed and cut into
quarters
¼ pound tiny green beans, trimmed
1 cup fresh or frozen corn kernels
1 small red bell pepper, cored, seeded, and cut into 1-inch squares
1 medium cucumber, seeded and cut into 1-inch cubes
2 large plum tomatoes, seeded and cut into 1-inch cubes
2 tablespoons chopped fresh basil or 2 teaspoons crushed dried
1 tablespoon fresh lemon juice
freshly ground pepper to taste

To make the yogurt cheese, place the yogurt in a fine strainer lined with a paper coffee filter or cheesecloth and position the strainer over a bowl. Cover and refrigerate overnight or for at least 8 hours. Remove the strained yogurt from the filter and place in a container. Discard the remaining liquid. Cover and refrigerate the yogurt cheese; you should have about 2 cups.

To make the soup, in a large pot, combine the water, vinegar, onion, and garlic. Bring to a boil over medium-high heat. Boil, covered, for 5 minutes. Add the potatoes, cover the pot, and continue to cook for another 10 minutes. Add the green beans, corn, and bell pepper. Cover and cook for another 1 to 2 minutes. Remove from the stove and cool to room temperature, then cover and refrigerate until thoroughly chilled, at least 3 hours.

When ready to serve, add the yogurt cheese to the cold vegetable mixture, slowly beating with a large wire whisk. Stir in the cucumber, tomatoes, basil, and lemon juice. Ladle into shallow soup bowls and season with pepper.

Makes 4 servings.

JOSLIN CHOICES: I very-low-fat protein, 2 carbohydrate (bread/starch), I vegetable
PER SERVING: 233 calories (3% calories from fat), I g total fat (0 saturated fat), 14 g protein,
45 g carbohydrates, 5 g dietary fiber, 3 mg cholesterol, 99 mg sodium, 1,174 mg potassium
JOSLIN CHOICES (yogurt cheese only): I carbohydrate (skim milk)
PER ½-CUP SERVING: 86 calories (19% calories from fat), 0 total fat (0 saturated fat), 9 g
protein, 12 g carbohydrates, 0 dietary fiber, 3 mg cholesterol, 86 mg sodium, 289 mg
potassium

Bean and Pasta Soup

This yummy version of *pasta e fagioli* is one of the most satisfying soups that we've tasted. You don't have to be Italian to love this soup, but when you enjoy it with a loaf of crusty Italian bread, some low-fat Italian cheese, and sliced pears, you may want to become an honorary Italian for the day.

1 tablespoon olive oil
1 rib celery, chopped
1 medium onion, coarsely chopped
2 large cloves garlic, minced
4 ounces dried cannellini beans, rinsed and picked over
1 small bay leaf
1 teaspoon crushed dried basil
½ teaspoon crushed dried thyme
⅛ teaspoon crushed dried rosemary
2 cups canned low-fat, low-sodium chicken or vegetable broth
3 cups water
1 14½-ounce can no-salt-added tomatoes with juice
2 ounces very small cut tubular pasta, such as ditali
salt to taste (optional)
freshly ground pepper to taste
1 ounce Parmigiano-Reggiano cheese
¼ cup lightly packed small fresh basil leaves

In a large pot, heat the oil over medium-low heat. Add the celery, onion, and garlic. Sauté, stirring occasionally, until the vegetables are limp, about 5 minutes. Stir in the beans, bay leaf, basil, thyme, rosemary, broth, water, and tomatoes. Cook, covered, over low heat until the beans are tender, about 1½ to 2 hours.

When the beans are soft, remove the bay leaf and add the pasta, salt (if using), and pepper. Cook for another 10 to 15 minutes, until the pasta is done.

Ladle into wide soup bowls. Using a vegetable peeler, shave cheese over each serving. Sprinkle with basil leaves and serve at once.

Makes 4 servings.

JOSLIN CHOICES: 1½ very-low-fat protein, 2 carbohydrate (bread/starch), 1 fat

PER SERVING: 246 calories (24% calories from fat), 7 g total fat (2 g saturated fat), 13 g protein, 35 g carbohydrates, 7 g dietary fiber, 7 mg cholesterol, 142 mg sodium, 651 mg potassium

Flemish Puree of Vegetable Soup

This soup has a sweet, rich, complex flavor that makes it perfect to serve to anyone who complains about eating vegetables. It is elegant enough to serve at a dinner party, yet easy enough to make anytime. When fresh pumpkins are available, try substituting a baby pumpkin (about 6 to 8 ounces) for the carrots. You won't be disappointed.

butter-flavored cooking spray
2 leeks, white part only, cut in half and rinsed well, thinly sliced
1 medium onion, chopped
4 cups canned low-fat, low-sodium chicken or vegetable broth
2 medium carrots, sliced into ½-inch-thick coins
1 medium russet potato, peeled and cut into 1-inch cubes
1 bay leaf
1 tablespoon fresh thyme leaves or 1 teaspoon crushed dried
½ cup skim milk
freshly ground pepper to taste
flat-leaf parsley for garnish

Coat a large nonstick pot with cooking spray. Add the leeks and onion; sauté until soft, about 4 minutes. Add the broth, carrots, potato, bay leaf, and thyme. Bring to a boil. Turn down the heat and simmer until the potatoes and carrots are tender, about 15 minutes. Remove and discard the bay leaf.

Puree the soup in batches in a food processor fitted with a metal blade or in a blender. Return the soup to the pot and stir in the milk and pepper. When ready to serve, reheat, ladle into bowls, and garnish with parsley.

Makes 6 servings.

JOSLIN CHOICES: 1 carbohydrate (bread/starch)

PER SERVING: 84 calories (13% calories from fat), 1 g total fat (1 g saturated fat), 4 g protein, 15 g carbohydrates, 2 g dietary fiber, 3 mg cholesterol, 98 mg sodium, 281 mg potassium

Spinach and Yogurt Soup

This is a filling soup to have with a sandwich for a quick meal. If you happen to grow sorrel or can buy it at your market, try it in place of the spinach for a different but equally delicious soup.

olive oil cooking spray
1 onion, chopped
1 10-ounce package frozen leaf spinach, thawed and well drained
1 cup water
2 cups plain nonfat yogurt
¼ teaspoon grated nutmeg
2 teaspoons fresh thyme or ½ teaspoon crushed dried
¾ cup canned low-fat, low-sodium chicken or vegetable broth
freshly ground pepper to taste
thyme sprigs for garnish

Lightly coat a nonstick pot with cooking spray and add the onion. Cook over medium heat until soft, about 4 minutes. Add the spinach and water. Raise the heat to high and cook until the water has evaporated. Remove from the heat. Stir in the yogurt, nutmeg, and thyme.

Puree the mixture in batches in a food processor fitted with a metal blade or in a blender. Return to the pot and stir in the broth. Season with pepper. Reheat but do not allow soup to boil.

Ladle into soup bowls and garnish with thyme.

Makes 4 servings.

JOSLIN CHOICES: ½ carbohydrate (½ nonfat milk), 1 vegetable
PER SERVING: 93 calories (5% calories from fat), 1 g total fat (0 saturated fat), 9 g protein, 16 g carbohydrates, 3 g dietary fiber, 3 mg cholesterol, 152 mg sodium, 46 mg potassium

Italian Pantry Soup with Basil-Roasted Tomatoes

*W*e call this a "pantry" soup because it uses a small amount of the many staples in your carbohydrate pantry, along with some vegetables you probably have on hand. All you need from your supermarket or garden is some fresh basil. The result is a hearty, delicious soup that can be served as a meal or in small portions as a first course.

BASIL-ROASTED TOMATOES
olive oil cooking spray
24 large fresh basil leaves, washed
8 medium plum tomatoes, cut in half lengthwise
1 tablespoon olive oil
freshly ground pepper to taste

SOUP
2 tablespoons dried lentils, rinsed and picked over
2 tablespoons dried split peas, rinsed and picked over
2 tablespoons dried small white beans, rinsed and picked over
8 cups canned low-fat, low-sodium chicken or vegetable broth
1 cup diced onion
½ cup diced celery
3 ounces small dried pasta, such as ditalini or tiny shells
¼ cup freshly grated Parmesan cheese

Preheat the oven to 450ºF.

With cooking spray, lightly coat a shallow baking dish large enough to hold the tomato halves in a single layer. Line the dish with the basil leaves and top with the tomato halves, cut side down. Drizzle with the olive oil and season with pepper. Bake, uncovered, for 1 hour, until the tomatoes are very tender. Remove from the oven and set aside.

Meanwhile, to make the soup, combine the lentils, split peas, and white beans in a large heavy saucepan. Add the broth and bring to a boil. Reduce the heat to a simmer, cover, and cook for 20 minutes. Add the onion and celery. Partially cover and cook for another 20 minutes. Stir in the pasta and continue to cook, uncovered, for another 7 to 8 minutes, until the pasta is tender.

Stir in the reserved tomato-basil mixture and cook until the tomatoes are heated through, about 5 minutes. Ladle into shallow soup bowls and garnish each serving with some of the Parmesan cheese. Serve at once.

Makes 6 main dish or 12 starter servings.

JOSLIN CHOICES: I medium-fat protein, I carbohydrate (bread/starch), I vegetable
PER MAIN DISH SERVING: 196 calories (27% calories from fat), 6 g total fat (2 g saturated
    fat), 12 g protein, 26 g carbohydrates, 6 g dietary fiber, 8 mg cholesterol, 241 mg sodium,
    429 mg potassium
JOSLIN CHOICES: I carbohydrate (bread/starch)
PER STARTER SERVING: 98 calories (27% calories from fat), 3 g total fat (I g saturated fat),
    6 g protein, 13 g carbohydrates, 3 g dietary fiber, 4 mg cholesterol, 120 mg sodium, 214 mg
    potassium

Herb-Roasted Tomato Soup

*G*rady Spears serves a terrific tomato soup at his popular Fort Worth restaurant, Reata, which is affiliated with and named after the Texas ranch on which the famous 1956 movie *Giant* was filmed. Grady has found that adding a bit of baking soda to fresh tomato soup reduces the acidity of the tomatoes, giving the soup a mild flavor. Our version is similar to the restaurant's—perfect for warding off winter chills or a summer cold.

olive oil cooking spray
6 large plum tomatoes (about 1½ pounds total), cut in half lengthwise
4 large cloves garlic, minced
1 small red onion, chopped
1 small red bell pepper, seeded and chopped
2 teaspoons crushed dried thyme
¼ teaspoon crushed dried basil
½ teaspoon salt (optional)

1 teaspoon freshly ground pepper
2 tablespoons balsamic vinegar
1 teaspoon brown sugar
¾ cup low-sodium tomato juice
¼ cup low-sodium tomato paste
½ teaspoon baking soda
1½ cups evaporated skim milk
¼ cup chopped fresh basil

Preheat the oven to 350°F. Lightly coat a medium baking pan with cooking spray.

Arrange the tomato halves in a single layer, cut side down, in the prepared pan. Top with the garlic, red onion, bell pepper, thyme, basil, salt (if using), pepper, balsamic vinegar, and brown sugar. Cover with aluminum foil and roast for 30 minutes, until the vegetables are very tender.

Transfer the vegetables to a food processor fitted with a metal blade. Process until smooth. Pour into a large saucepan. Add the tomato juice, tomato paste, and baking soda. Mix well. Add the evaporated skim milk and simmer for 20 minutes to allow the flavors to thoroughly blend.

Ladle into hot soup bowls. Sprinkle each serving with basil and serve.

Makes 4 servings.

JOSLIN CHOICES: 2 carbohydrate (1 bread/starch, 1 nonfat milk)
PER SERVING: 164 calories (5% calories from fat), 1 g total fat (0 saturated fat), 10 g protein,
   31 g carbohydrates, 4 g dietary fiber, 3 mg cholesterol, 619 mg sodium, 957 mg potassium

Sun-Dried Tomato and Lentil Soup

This delicious soup not only is beautiful in the bowl, with its contrast of pink lentils, red tomatoes, and green basil, but is so quick and easy to make that you can have it ready in less than 30 minutes, making it perfect for a light supper after a long day.

olive oil cooking spray
1 medium onion, chopped

1 large clove garlic, minced
1 cup dried red lentils, rinsed and picked over
½ cup dry-packed sun-dried tomatoes, chopped
4 cups canned low-fat, low-sodium chicken or vegetable broth
freshly ground pepper to taste
¼ cup chopped fresh basil
¼ cup fat-free sour cream

Coat a nonstick pot with cooking spray. Add the onion and sauté over medium heat until soft. Add the garlic and sauté for 1 minute more. Add the lentils, sun-dried tomatoes, and broth. Bring to a boil, lower the heat, and simmer for 20 minutes. Stir in the pepper and basil.

Divide the soup among 4 bowls and top each serving with sour cream. Serve immediately.

Makes 4 servings.

JOSLIN CHOICES: 1 very-low-fat protein, 2 carbohydrate (bread/starch)

PER SERVING: 228 calories (7% calories from fat), 2 g total fat (1 g saturated fat), 16 g
    protein, 38 g carbohydrates, 8 g dietary fiber, 5 mg cholesterol, 278 mg sodium, 685 mg
    potassium

Tortilla Soup

*A*lmost every restaurant seems to have a version of tortilla soup. This recipe is inspired by one of the best we've tasted. At a popular diner in San Francisco, the soup was made without the customary strips of chicken, but the combination was so flavorful that the chicken was never missed.

4 medium fresh tomatoes (about 1½ pounds total), quartered
1 medium onion, quartered
vegetable cooking spray
6 7-inch corn tortillas
6 large cloves garlic, finely chopped

8 cups canned low-fat, low-sodium chicken or vegetable broth
¼ cup low-sodium tomato paste
1 tablespoon chopped fresh cilantro
1 tablespoon ground cumin
½ tablespoon good-quality chili powder
2 small bay leaves
salt to taste (optional)
1 small ripe avocado, peeled and diced
⅓ cup shredded reduced-fat cheddar cheese

In a food processor fitted with a metal blade, puree the tomatoes and onion until smooth. Set aside.

Lightly coat the bottom of a large nonstick saucepan with cooking spray. Coarsely chop 3 tortillas and add to the pan with the garlic; sauté for 2 to 3 minutes. Add the tomato-onion mixture, chicken stock, tomato paste, cilantro, cumin, chili powder, and bay leaves. Bring to a boil; reduce the heat, cover, and simmer for 30 minutes. Remove and discard the bay leaves. Season with salt (if using).

While the soup is cooking, preheat the oven to 350°F.

Cut the remaining 3 tortillas in half, then into 2-inch-wide strips. Spread the tortilla strips in a single layer on a large baking sheet. Bake for 10 to 12 minutes, shaking the pan occasionally, until the strips are crisp. Remove from the oven and set aside.

To serve, ladle the soup into 6 soup bowls. Top each serving with some of the tortilla strips, avocado, and a scant tablespoon of shredded cheese. Serve at once.

Makes 6 servings.

JOSLIN CHOICES: I very-low-fat protein, I carbohydrate (bread/starch), I vegetable, I fat
PER SERVING: 219 calories (35% calories from fat), 9 g total fat (2 g saturated fat), 10 g
protein, 28 g carbohydrates, 5 g dietary fiber, 6 mg cholesterol, 250 mg sodium, 677 mg
potassium

Soupe au Pistou

Welcome to the south of France! If this soup tastes a lot like Italy, it is because the two Mediterranean countries are close enough in proximity and culture to share the love of basil, fresh vegetables, pasta, and cheese. Pistou is France's version of Italy's beloved pesto sauce.

Soupe au Pistou is wonderful the day it is made, but it's just as good—some say even better—the next, so feel free to make extra to store in the refrigerator for a couple of days or to freeze for up to 2 months.

olive oil cooking spray
1 large onion, chopped
2 large cloves garlic, minced
1 15-ounce can cannellini beans, rinsed well and drained
2 small russet potatoes, peeled and diced
1 medium carrot, diced
2 small zucchini, sliced
1 14½-ounce can no-salt-added diced tomatoes
2 tablespoons chopped fresh basil
4 cups canned low-fat, low-sodium chicken or vegetable broth
2 ounces small dried pasta (your choice of shape)

PISTOU
2 tablespoons grated Parmesan cheese
1 tablespoon pine nuts
3 tablespoons chopped fresh basil
2 large cloves garlic
1 tablespoon olive oil
⅛ teaspoon freshly ground pepper

Coat a large nonstick pot with cooking spray. Add the onion and sauté over medium heat until softened. Add the garlic, beans, potatoes, carrot, zucchini, tomatoes, and basil. Cook over medium heat for 3 to 4 minutes, stirring occasionally. Pour in the stock, cover, and simmer for 20 to 25 minutes.

Meanwhile, make the pistou. Place all the ingredients in a food processor fitted with a metal blade or in a blender, and process until smooth.

Add the pasta to the soup and simmer, uncovered, until it is cooked al dente, about 8 to 10 minutes. Ladle into bowls and top with a teaspoon of pistou.

Makes 4 servings.

JOSLIN CHOICES: 1 low-fat protein, 3 carbohydrate (bread/starch), 1 fat

PER SERVING: 345 calories (21% calories from fat), 8 g total fat (2 g saturated fat), 15 g
protein, 55 g carbohydrates, 9 g dietary fiber, 6 mg cholesterol, 412 mg sodium, 865 mg
potassium

Vegetable Chili

What do you get when you mix hot and spicy Tex-Mex chili with stewed vegetables? You get a lunch or dinner that will make your taste buds come alive. Serve this chili with homemade baked corn chips, sliced pickled okra, chopped onion, fat-free sour cream, and grated reduced-fat cheddar cheese for a meal that will be met with *Olé!*

olive oil cooking spray
1 medium onion, chopped
2 large cloves garlic, minced
1 tablespoon chili powder
1 tablespoon ground cumin
2 14½-ounce cans no-salt-added tomatoes, chopped with juice
1 15-ounce can red kidney beans, rinsed well
1 large green bell pepper, seeded and chopped into ½-inch dice
1 large red bell pepper, seeded and chopped into ½-inch dice
1 jalapeño chile pepper, seeded and minced
2 small zucchini, quartered and sliced
2 small yellow summer squash, quartered and sliced
1 large ear fresh corn, shucked and silk removed, cut crosswise into 6 pieces
3 tablespoons chopped fresh cilantro
freshly ground pepper to taste

Lightly coat a large nonstick pot with cooking spray and add the onion. Cook over medium heat until the onion is limp, about 4 minutes. Add the garlic and sauté for 1 minute. Stir in the chili powder and cumin. Stir and cook for another minute.

Add the tomatoes, beans, bell peppers, chile pepper, zucchini, summer squash, and corn. Cover and simmer for 30 minutes. Add the cilantro and season with pepper. Ladle into soup bowls, putting 1 corn piece into each bowl. Serve immediately.

Makes 6 servings.

JOSLIN CHOICES: 1 very-low-fat protein, 1½ carbohydrate (bread/starch)
PER SERVING: 188 calories (7% calories from fat), 1 g total fat (0 saturated fat), 10 g protein, 37 g carbohydrates, 13 g dietary fiber, 0 cholesterol, 225 mg sodium, 881 mg potassium

Curried Cauliflower Stew

*N*othing brightens the day like the aroma of a good curry cooking. Serve this one with basmati rice flavored with a tablespoon each of toasted slivered almonds and currants plumped first in a bit of dry sherry.

vegetable cooking spray
1 large onion, thinly sliced
2½-inch piece fresh ginger, peeled and minced
1 teaspoon ground cumin
1 to 1½ teaspoons curry powder, to taste
1 large head cauliflower (about 1½ pounds), florets cut into bite-size pieces
1 medium red apple, unpeeled, cored and chopped
¾ cup canned low-fat, low-sodium chicken or vegetable broth
½ teaspoon kosher salt (optional)
1 10-ounce package frozen baby peas
1 teaspoon garam masala (recipe follows)

Lightly coat a nonstick covered pot with cooking spray. Add the onion and cook over medium heat until softened, about 4 minutes. Add the ginger, cumin, and curry powder; stir for 2 minutes.

Stir in the cauliflower and coat with the spices. Add the apple, broth, and salt (if using). Cover and simmer for about 8 to 10 minutes, until the vegetables and apple are cooked through. Add the peas and bring to a boil. Lower the heat and simmer for 2 minutes. Sprinkle with garam masala and continue to simmer until the peas are heated through. Serve hot.

Makes 4 servings.

JOSLIN CHOICES: ½ very-low-fat protein, 1 carbohydrate (bread/starch)
PER SERVING: 125 calories (7% calories from fat), 1 g total fat (0 saturated fat), 7 g protein,
    25 g carbohydrates, 8 g dietary fiber, 1 mg cholesterol, 533 mg sodium, 634 mg potassium

Garam Masala

Garam masala is available in specialty stores, or you can follow this simple recipe to make your own.

1 tablespoon cardamom seeds
1 tablespoon coriander seeds
1 tablespoon cumin seeds
1 teaspoon black peppercorns
½ teaspoon whole cloves
2 teaspoons ground cinnamon
¼ teaspoon ground nutmeg

Place the cardamom, coriander, cumin, peppercorns, and cloves in a small skillet and cook over low heat until fragrant. Cool and grind in a spice grinder or mortar and pestle. Add the cinnamon and nutmeg. Store in an airtight container.

Makes about 3 tablespoons.

Fennel, Tomato, and Cannellini Stew

The earthy flavors of Mediterranean food shine in this stew. Serve it with garlic crostini and follow with some fresh fruit, rich coffee, and Lemon Biscotti (page 221) alongside. You will be transported abroad.

olive oil cooking spray
2 leeks, white part only, halved and washed well, chopped
3 cloves garlic, minced
1 large bulb fennel, halved, cored, and thinly sliced
2 cups canned low-fat, low-sodium chicken or vegetable broth
1 28-ounce can no-salt-added Italian tomatoes with their juice
5 sprigs fresh thyme
2 small bay leaves
freshly ground pepper to taste
2 15-ounce cans cannellini beans, rinsed well

GARLIC CROSTINI
1 thin baguette (about 1 pound), cut into ⅓-inch-thick slices
2 large cloves garlic, halved

Lightly coat a large nonstick covered pot with cooking spray. Sauté the leeks over medium heat until wilted, about 5 minutes. Add the garlic and fennel; continue to cook for 2 minutes. Pour in the broth and tomatoes. With the back of a wooden spoon, break the tomatoes into pieces. Bring to a boil and add the thyme, bay leaves, and pepper. Cover and simmer for 15 to 20 minutes, until the vegetables are soft. Add the beans and cook until heated through.

To make the crostini, toast or grill both sides of the bread. While still warm, rub each side with garlic cloves.

To serve, discard the thyme sprigs and bay leaves. Ladle the soup into individual bowls and top each serving with 2 slices of crostini.

Makes 8 servings.

JOSLIN CHOICES: 4 carbohydrate (bread/starch), 1 fat

PER SERVING: 377 calories (16% calories from fat), 7 g total fat (1 g saturated fat), 11 g protein, 68 g carbohydrates, 11 g dietary fiber, 1 mg cholesterol, 617 mg sodium, 531 mg potassium

Gardener's Stew in a Ring of Wild Rice

*H*ere we've used a ring of cooked wild rice, studded with dried cherries and flavored with orange zest and herbs, to serve as a holder for a savory vegetable stew that's chock-full of garden-fresh vegetables. For more about wild rice, see page 166.

RICE RING
4 cups water
1 cup wild rice, rinsed and drained
olive oil cooking spray
1 small onion, chopped
1 rib celery, chopped
¼ cup chopped dried cherries
1 tablespoon grated orange zest
1 teaspoon crushed dried thyme
½ teaspoon crushed dried sage

STEW
2 medium onions, chopped
2 large cloves garlic, minced
1 large green bell pepper, seeded and coarsely chopped
1 small Japanese eggplant, unpeeled, cut into 2-inch cubes
2 medium yellow summer squash, halved lengthwise and cut into 2-inch-thick slices
3 medium tomatoes, coarsely chopped
¼ cup chopped flat-leaf parsley
½ cup low-sodium vegetable juice
1 tablespoon low-sodium tomato paste
1 teaspoon crushed dried thyme
salt to taste (optional)

freshly ground pepper to taste
½ cup frozen peas, thawed

In a large saucepan, bring the water to a rapid boil. Add the rice, reduce the heat, and simmer, uncovered, over medium-low heat until just tender, 30 to 45 minutes. Do not overcook. When done, drain and fluff with a fork. Set aside.

Meanwhile, lightly coat a large nonstick skillet with cooking spray. Add the onion and celery and place over medium-high heat. Sauté, stirring occasionally, until the vegetables wilt, about 5 minutes. Stir in the dried cherries, orange zest, thyme, and sage. Set aside.

To prepare the stew, lightly coat a second large nonstick skillet with cooking spray. Place over medium heat and add the onions and garlic. Sauté until the onions wilt, about 5 minutes. Add the bell pepper, eggplant, summer squash, tomatoes, and parsley.

In a measuring cup, whisk together the vegetable juice, tomato paste, and thyme. Pour over the vegetables and stir well. Taste and season with salt (if using) and pepper. Partially cover and let the stew simmer for 20 to 25 minutes, until the vegetables are tender and the flavors have blended. During the last 5 minutes of cooking time, stir in the peas.

To mold the rice, lightly coat an 8-inch ring mold with cooking spray. Stir the reserved wild rice into the onion-cherry mixture and reheat gently, stirring occasionally. Tightly pack the hot rice mixture in the prepared ring mold. Invert onto a large serving plate and remove the mold.

Immediately fill the center with the hot vegetable stew, spooning any pan juices over the vegetables. Serve at once.

Makes 4 servings.

JOSLIN CHOICES: 4 carbohydrate (bread/starch)
PER SERVING: 343 calories (4% calories from fat), 2 g total fat (0 saturated fat), 13 g protein, 74 g carbohydrates, 14 g dietary fiber, 0 cholesterol, 76 mg sodium, 1,289 mg potassium

Potato and Eggplant Stew

*T*his vegetable stew is evocative of the French countryside. Add crusty bread and a salad studded with chopped Niçoise olives and ripe tomatoes, and you have a quickly made, substantial meal.

> *1 large eggplant (about 1 pound)*
> *⅛ teaspoon kosher salt*
> *olive oil cooking spray*
> *1 large onion, chopped*
> *1 8-ounce package fresh button mushrooms, cleaned and halved*
> *1 large russet potato, peeled and cut into ¾-inch cubes*
> *½ teaspoon crushed dried herbes de Provence*
> *⅛ teaspoon salt (optional)*
> *freshly ground pepper to taste*

Cut the eggplant in half lengthwise, score it, and sprinkle with the kosher salt. After 20 minutes, wipe off the eggplant juice and salt with paper towels. Peel the eggplant and cut into 1-inch cubes.

Lightly coat a nonstick pot with cooking spray. Add the onion and cook over medium heat until softened, about 5 minutes. Add the mushrooms, potato, eggplant, and herbs. Cover and simmer for 12 to 15 minutes, until the vegetables are tender. Taste and season with salt (if using) and pepper. Serve hot.

Makes 4 servings.

JOSLIN CHOICES: 1 carbohydrate (bread/starch)
PER SERVING: 94 calories (5% calories from fat), 1 g total fat (0 saturated fat), 3 g protein, 21 g carbohydrates, 4 g dietary fiber, 0 cholesterol, 140 mg sodium, 690 mg potassium

Slow-Roasted Vegetable Stew

*A*lmost any vegetable except leafy greens can be roasted to bring out its natural sugars. Here a delicious assortment of vegetables is roasted, then interspersed at the last minute with wilted Swiss chard for an attractive table presentation.

1 small butternut squash (about 1 pound), peeled and cut into 2-inch wedges

6 small carrots, peeled, leaving ¼ inch of green tops attached

3 small red bell peppers, seeded and cut into quarters lengthwise

1 small bulb fennel, white part only, quartered

12 small white boiling onions, peeled

6 small plum tomatoes, stem end removed and halved lengthwise

1 tablespoon olive oil

2 tablespoons chopped flat-leaf parsley

1 tablespoon fresh thyme leaves or 1 teaspoon crushed dried

salt to taste (optional)

freshly ground pepper to taste

olive oil cooking spray

1 large clove garlic, peeled and thinly sliced

½ pound greens, such as Swiss chard, mustard, or spinach, washed

balsamic vinegar

2 ounces Parmesan cheese, freshly shaved or grated

¼ cup chopped fresh basil (optional)

Preheat the oven to 400°F.

Arrange the squash, carrots, bell peppers, fennel, onions, and tomatoes in a large roasting pan. Drizzle with the olive oil and sprinkle with the parsley and thyme. Season with salt (if using) and pepper. Roast, uncovered, for 20 minutes. Turn the vegetables and continue to roast for another 20 to 30 minutes, until all are tender.

Just as the vegetables are done, lightly coat a nonstick skillet with cooking spray. Place over medium-high heat. Add the garlic slices and sauté for 1 minute. Add the still damp greens and stir-fry for 1 to 2 minutes, until the greens are wilted. Sprinkle with balsamic vinegar.

To serve, spoon the vegetables and their broth into shallow soup bowls. Add 2 or

3 clumps of the braised greens and sprinkle with the shaved cheese. Sprinkle the basil (if using) over all and serve immediately.

Makes 4 servings.

JOSLIN CHOICES: ½ very-low-fat protein, 3 carbohydrate (bread/starch), I vegetable, I fat
PER SERVING: 368 calories (21% calories from fat), 9 g total fat (3 g saturated fat), 15 g
   protein, 64 g carbohydrates, 15 g dietary fiber, I I mg cholesterol, 486 mg sodium, 2,160
   mg potassium

Winter Vegetable Stew

*A*lthough we live in mild areas of the country, it sometimes seems as if winter will never end—with cold, drizzly days and a bitter wind blowing from the north. That's when vegetable stews are most welcome. They smell wonderful while they're cooking, and eating them warms you from the inside out.

To make this stew attractive, cut the vegetables in large pieces. For color we use plenty of carrots and vine-ripened organic plum tomatoes, which we can get all winter.

4 small carrots, peeled and cut in half crosswise
2 medium parsnips, peeled, cut in half lengthwise, then cut into 3-inch pieces
2 small turnips, peeled and quartered
4 medium ribs celery, cut into thirds
2 medium leeks, white part only, well rinsed and cut into thirds
1 medium onion, peeled and cut into eighths
2 large cloves garlic, peeled and quartered
1 small sweet potato, peeled and quartered
8 small button mushrooms, cleaned
4 medium ripe plum tomatoes, halved lengthwise
1 fresh lemon, washed and quartered, seeds removed
6 sprigs flat-leaf parsley
1 small bay leaf
1½ cups dry white wine or canned low-fat, low-sodium chicken or vegetable broth

1 tablespoon fresh thyme leaves or 1 teaspoon crushed dried
½ medium cabbage (about ½ pound), cored and quartered

Preheat the oven to 375ºF.

Arrange the carrots, parsnips, turnips, celery, leeks, onion, garlic, sweet potato, mushrooms, and plum tomatoes in a large oven-to-table baking dish. Add the lemon quarters, parsley, and bay leaf. Pour the wine or broth over the vegetables and sprinkle with the thyme.

Cover and bake for 45 minutes. Uncover and add the cabbage. Baste the vegetables and cabbage with pan juices. Cover and continue to bake for another 15 minutes, until the cabbage is tender. Discard the lemon, parsley, and bay leaf. To serve, spoon the vegetables into shallow soup bowls.

Makes 4 servings.

JOSLIN CHOICES: 2 carbohydrate (bread/starch), 2 vegetable
PER SERVING: 227 calories (8% calories from fat), 2 g total fat (1 g saturated fat), 8 g protein, 52 g carbohydrates, 12 g dietary fiber, 1 mg cholesterol, 163 mg sodium, 1,378 mg potassium

Lentil Burgers

Serve these tasty lentil burgers with fresh salsa or on a whole wheat bun with mustard, lettuce, and tomato. They freeze well, so they can be made ahead of time, frozen, then cooked directly from the freezer, giving you a quick meal whenever you want one.

1 cup dried green or brown lentils, rinsed and picked over
2 small onions
1 bay leaf
2 cups water
vegetable cooking spray
2 carrots, grated
6 ounces fresh mushrooms, chopped
2 cloves garlic, minced
1 teaspoon ground cumin
1 teaspoon chili powder
½ teaspoon salt (optional)
freshly ground pepper to taste
unbleached flour for coating
1 teaspoon canola oil

Place the lentils in a covered pot along with 1 onion cut in half and the bay leaf. Add the water and bring to a boil. Lower the heat to a simmer, cover, and cook for about 15 minutes, until the lentils are soft. Drain well, remove the bay leaf and onion, and set aside.

Coat a nonstick skillet with cooking spray. Chop the remaining onion into medium dice and add to the pan. Cook for 1 minute and then add the carrots and mushrooms. Sauté for 4 minutes, until soft. Add the garlic and cook another 2 to 3 minutes. Stir in the cumin and chili powder and coat the vegetables.

Combine the lentils and vegetables in the bowl of a food processor fitted with a metal blade. Season with the salt (if using) and pepper. Pulse the processor until the mixture begins to hold together. Leave small pieces of lentils and vegetables for texture.

With floured hands, form patties using ½ cup of the lentil mixture for each patty. Place on a floured piece of waxed paper. Continue until you use all of the mixture. Dust the tops with some extra flour.

Coat a large nonstick skillet with cooking spray and add the oil. Sauté the burgers over medium-high heat until brown. Carefully turn to brown the other side. Serve immediately.

Makes 8 servings.

JOSLIN CHOICES: 1 carbohydrate (bread/starch)
PER SERVING: 104 calories (7% calories from fat), 1 g total fat (0 saturated fat), 6 g protein,
    18 g carbohydrates, 5 g dietary fiber, 0 cholesterol, 164 mg sodium, 357 mg potassium

VARIATIONS

◆ Substitute dried thyme and sage for the cumin and chili powder. Serve with caramelized onion rings.
◆ Substitute fresh ginger and dried tandoori mix powder for the cumin and chili powder. Serve with a yogurt sauce seasoned with fresh cilantro and garlic.
◆ Substitute Worcestershire sauce and a bit of Dijon mustard for the cumin and chili powder. Serve with sliced fresh tomatoes, lettuce leaves, and dill pickle slices.

Grilled Portobello Mushroom Burger

*P*ortobellos have a rich, meaty flavor and grill so quickly that a portobello burger can appeal as much as a good old-fashioned hamburger. Here we serve it open-faced on a slice of grilled peasant-style bread, but you could tuck it into a hamburger bun.

4 portobello mushroom caps, about 5 inches in diameter
1 tablespoon olive oil
4 thin slices red onion
4 ounces thinly sliced skim milk Swiss cheese
4 teaspoons Dijon mustard
4 slices peasant-style bread
salt to taste (optional)
freshly ground pepper to taste
1 cup alfalfa sprouts or coarsely chopped watercress leaves

Light a grill or preheat the broiler.

Rinse and dry the mushrooms. Lightly rub with the olive oil. Grill, gill sides down, over hot coals or broil until the mushrooms start to release their juices, about 5 minutes.

Turn the mushrooms over and continue to grill until they are flexible when pressed, about 5 to 7 minutes.

Lay a slice of red onion on each cap and cover with cheese. Continue cooking until the cheese melts, about 3 minutes.

Meanwhile, brush the mustard on one side of each slice of bread. Place, mustard side down, on the grill until lightly toasted, about 2 minutes. Turn and toast the other side.

To serve, place a piece of toasted bread, mustard side up, on each of 4 plates. Set a mushroom burger on each bread slice. Season with salt (if using) and pepper. Top with some of the sprouts and serve at once.

Makes 4 servings.

JOSLIN CHOICES: 1½ low-fat protein, 1 carbohydrate (bread/starch), 1 fat
PER SERVING: 217 calories (44% calories from fat), 11 g total fat (5 g saturated fat), 14 g
  protein, 18 g carbohydrates, 5 g dietary fiber, 20 mg cholesterol, 390 mg sodium, 101 mg
  potassium

Low-Fat Cheese

*Y*ears ago cheese was a high-fat food, but today most markets are full of low-fat and fat-free choices. Choosing a low-fat or fat-free cheese requires extra care in selection and cooking.

First, read the labels carefully. Then try the different cheeses that your market offers. Brands are not all the same. We've found excellent brands of low-fat ricotta, mozzarella, cheddar, Swiss, cottage cheese, goat cheese, feta cheese, and cream cheese.

Low-fat cheese melts in the same way as mild cheeses but will toughen if a toaster, broiler, or direct heat is used. Low-fat cheese melts best with low heat, so if using in a sauce, stir in only one direction, adding a smidgen of flour or cornstarch to the shredded cheese before adding to the sauce. Fat-free cheese, on the other hand, doesn't melt smoothly but is excellent served cold, or it can be used in cooking with some change in texture and loss in taste. You can also mix low-fat and fat-free cheeses when cooking in order to reduce calories but still retain some of the melting capability and taste.

Quesadillas with Green Pea 'Mole

*W*e love quesadillas and often fix them for a quick lunch. Instead of the traditional guacamole accompaniment made with avocados, we make the dip with thawed frozen peas. Its pale green color is as lively as guacamole, and its tangy flavor complements the quesadilla without the added fat of the avocado. You will have extra; use the rest of the dip for an appetizer with fresh crudités within one day. And for those times when only the real thing will do, use Spicy Quacamole (page 99).

PER QUESADILLA
1 7-inch 98% fat-free flour tortilla
⅓ cup shredded skim milk Monterey Jack cheese
1 canned green chile, cut into thin strips

1 scallion, white part and 1 inch green, chopped
3 tablespoons Green Pea 'Mole (recipe follows)
1 tablespoon fat-free sour cream
1 teaspoon minced fresh cilantro, flat-leaf parsley, or mint

Preheat the oven to 350°F.

Lay the tortilla on a baking sheet. Spread the cheese over half of the tortilla and top with the chile strips and scallion. Fold the empty half over to cover the cheese and press down slightly. Brush the top of the tortilla lightly with water. Bake until crisp and the cheese is melted, about 12 minutes.

Cut the quesadilla into 3 triangles. Mound 3 tablespoons of the Green Pea 'Mole in the center of a serving plate. Surround with quesadilla triangles. Add a dollop of sour cream and sprinkle cilantro over all.

Makes 1 serving.

JOSLIN CHOICES: I low-fat protein, 2 carbohydrate (bread/starch), I vegetable
PER SERVING: 252 calories (13% calories from fat), 4 g total fat (I g saturated fat), 18 g protein, 35 g carbohydrates, 3 g dietary fiber, 9 mg cholesterol, 638 mg sodium, 221 mg potassium

Green Pea 'Mole

1 16-ounce bag frozen peas, thawed and drained
1 small onion, chopped
2 canned green chile peppers, coarsely chopped
1 tablespoon fresh lemon juice
½ teaspoon ground cumin

Place all the ingredients in a food processor fitted with a metal blade or in a blender. Process until smooth. Transfer to a covered container and refrigerate until ready to use.

Makes about 2½ cups.

JOSLIN CHOICES: I vegetable
PER (3-tablespoon) SERVING: 30 calories (5% calories from fat), 0 total fat (0 saturated fat), 2 g protein, 5 g carbohydrates, 2 g dietary fiber, 0 cholesterol, 47 mg sodium, 68 mg potassium

Spicy Guacamole

Since the fat of the avocado is monounsaturated, avocados can be included in a healthy meal plan, so sometimes we serve quesadillas with a traditional guacamole. We prefer guacamole to have a chunky texture, so we finely dice the avocado rather than making a puree in the blender or food processor.

For this recipe you'll need ripe Hass avocados (the dark-skinned ones from California). The large green avocados from Florida are more watery, with less flavor. If you wish, you can substitute fresh lemon juice and flat-leaf parsley for the fresh lime juice and cilantro.

½ cup chopped red onion
½ cup seeded and chopped ripe tomatoes
1 to 2 jalapeño chile peppers, seeded and minced (depending on your heat tolerance)
2 tablespoons chopped fresh cilantro
3 tablespoons fresh lime juice
3 ripe avocados, pitted and peeled
salt to taste (optional)
freshly ground pepper to taste

Place the onion, tomatoes, chile peppers, cilantro, and lime juice in a food processor. Pulse until finely minced.

Finely dice the avocados and gently fold in the tomato-onion mixture. Season with salt (if using) and pepper. Serve at once or tightly cover with plastic wrap and refrigerate for up to 1 hour before serving.

Makes 2½ cups.

JOSLIN CHOICES: 2 fat
PER ¼-CUP SERVING: 99 calories (76% calories from fat), 9 g total fat (1 g saturated fat), 1 g
    protein, 5 g carbohydrates, 3 g dietary fiber, 0 cholesterol, 7 mg sodium, 371 mg potassium

Grilled Tofu Sandwich

*T*his open-faced sandwich packs a lot of taste in each bite, thanks to the mustard marinade. It makes for a light lunch or dinner that will surprise you with its "meaty" taste.

MARINADE
2 cloves garlic, minced
2 scallions, white part only, minced
1 tablespoon Dijon mustard
2 tablespoons balsamic vinegar
2 tablespoons olive oil
⅛ teaspoon crushed red pepper flakes
⅛ teaspoon sugar substitute

8 ⅓-inch-thick slices (about 12 ounces) firm tofu, pressed and weighted down (see page 179)
1 tablespoon mayonnaise
1 teaspoon Dijon mustard
⅛ teaspoon prepared horseradish, or to taste
4 slices whole wheat bread
4 leaves Boston lettuce, washed and crisped
1 medium tomato, sliced into 4 slices
½ small sweet onion (such as Vidalia, Walla Walla, Maui, or Texas Sweet 1015), very thinly sliced

To make the marinade, combine the garlic, scallions, mustard, vinegar, oil, red pepper flakes, and sugar substitute in a small bowl.

Place the slices of drained and pressed tofu in a flat dish. Pour the marinade over the tofu and marinate for at least 1 hour or overnight, turning several times to coat both sides.

Light a grill or preheat the broiler.

Transfer the tofu slices to a paper towel to drain. Grill or broil on both sides until browned and the edges become slightly crisp.

Combine the mayonnaise, mustard, and horseradish. Spread 1 teaspoon of the mayonnaise mixture on each slice of bread. Top with the lettuce, tomato slices, and grilled tofu. Top with onion slices and serve at once.

Makes 4 servings.

JOSLIN CHOICES: 1 medium-fat protein, 1 carbohydrate (bread/starch), 1 vegetable, 2 fat
PER SERVING: 257 calories (50% calories from fat), 15 g total fat (2 g saturated fat), 11 g protein, 23 g carbohydrates, 3 g dietary fiber, 3 mg cholesterol, 307 mg sodium, 404 mg potassium

Veggie Sandwich

This is a favorite for lunch at our homes. Be sure to buy the best-quality multigrain bread and include plenty of sprouts. A seedless cucumber (sometimes labeled English or hothouse) is the long, slender cucumber that comes wrapped in plastic.

3 tablespoons reduced-calorie mayonnaise
1 teaspoon country-style Dijon mustard
8 slices dark multigrain bread
1 small avocado, peeled and pitted
2 teaspoons fresh lemon juice
4 ounces fat-free Swiss cheese, thinly sliced
1 medium red bell pepper, cored, seeded, and cut into thin rings
¼ seedless cucumber, peeled and thinly sliced on the diagonal
1 large ripe tomato, cut into 8 thin slices
freshly ground pepper to taste
2 teaspoons chopped fresh dill
½ cup alfalfa-radish sprouts

Combine the mayonnaise and mustard. Spread on one side of 4 bread slices. Set aside.

In a small bowl, mash the avocado with the lemon juice. Spread the avocado mixture on one side of the remaining 4 bread slices. Top each with 1 ounce of the Swiss cheese, 2 bell pepper rings, 2 to 3 cucumber slices, 2 slices of tomato, and a generous grinding of pepper.

Sprinkle each sandwich with ½ teaspoon of the chopped dill and arrange the sprouts on top. Cover with the reserved bread slices, mayonnaise side down. Cut in half and serve at once.

Makes 4 servings.

JOSLIN CHOICES: I very-low-fat protein, 2 carbohydrate (bread/starch), 2 fat
PER SERVING: 300 calories (35% calories from fat), 12 g total fat (2 g saturated fat), 14 g
protein, 37 g carbohydrates, 7 g dietary fiber, 3 mg cholesterol, 727 mg sodium, 692 mg
potassium

Stacked Cake Sandwich

*S*tacked tea sandwiches with their creamy and flavorful fillings have been staples of lovely tea tables on both sides of the Atlantic. Here we have taken the idea and improved it, making it low in fat, modern in taste, and even more beautiful to the eyes. Make this early in the day, then sit back and wait for your guests to be impressed.

3 ounces firm tofu, pressed and chopped fine
1 teaspoon chopped fresh chives
2 tablespoons fat-free mayonnaise
1 to 2 teaspoons Dijon mustard, to taste
freshly ground pepper to taste
1 large plum tomato, peeled, seeded, and finely diced
3 tablespoons hummus (page 33)
2 tablespoons fat-free sour cream
½ to 1 teaspoon prepared horseradish, to taste
½ teaspoon fresh lemon juice
1 1-pound loaf unsliced whole wheat bread, all crusts removed (see Note)
1 2-inch section seedless cucumber, very thinly sliced
1 16-ounce container nonfat cottage cheese, drained
extra chives, cucumber slices, tomato skin roses, fresh herb sprigs, and edible flowers,
such as nasturtiums, pansies, or violets, for garnish (optional)

Place the tofu, chives, mayonnaise, and mustard in a bowl and mix well. Season with pepper. Set aside.

Combine the tomato and hummus in a separate bowl until the tomato is coated. Season with pepper. Set aside.

Combine the sour cream, horseradish, and lemon juice in a third bowl. Set aside.

To assemble the sandwich, carefully slice the bread lengthwise with a very sharp knife into 4 long slices of equal thickness. Place the first slice on a serving platter and cover with the tofu filling. Cover with a second slice of bread. Spread with the hummus-tomato filling. Cover with a third piece of bread. Spread with the sour cream mixture and cover with overlapping slices of cucumber. Top with the last slice of bread.

Place the drained cottage cheese in a food processor fitted with a metal blade. Process until very smooth and creamy. Spread over the top and on the long sides of the sandwich stack, leaving the two ends unfrosted. Make a lattice with chives by criss-crossing them on top of the sandwich cake. Decorate the sides with cucumber slices, tomato skin roses, fresh herbs, and edible flowers. Refrigerate until ready to serve.

When ready to serve, cut a thin slice off the unfrosted ends to expose the fillings. Cut the remaining sandwich cake into ¾-inch-thick slices.

Makes 10 slices.

Note: If you can't find unsliced bread, use whole wheat bread slices with the crust removed. Place 2 next to each other for each layer. Do try to find bread that has body and texture rather than the overprocessed commercial kind.

JOSLIN CHOICES: 1 low-fat protein, 1 carbohydrate (bread/starch), 1 vegetable
PER 1-SLICE SERVING: 169 calories (16% calories from fat), 3 g total fat (1 g saturated fat),
    12 g protein, 25 g carbohydrates, 4 g dietary fiber, 4 mg cholesterol, 458 mg sodium,
    222 mg potassium

∼STUFFED PITA SANDWICHES∼

*P*ita bread, also known as pocket bread, makes preparing sandwiches easy, as the rounds split easily and beg to be filled with a variety of savory fillings. Here we give you three delicious fillings, but let your imagination go and you'll think of many more.

Grilled Vegetable Pitas

*M*any vegetables profit from grilling. Depending on what you have in your refrigerator, this sandwich will change, but the raves you get when you serve it won't. You'll need to parboil the fennel and potatoes until just about done, then slice, brush with the marinade, and grill. That way they will be done at the same time as the other vegetables.

We've found that when stuffing a pita sandwich, you can prevent it from tearing so easily while eating if you cut each pita in half, carefully open each half, then insert one half (open side out) inside the second. This gives you a much stronger pocket of bread to hold the stuffing.

MARINADE
2 tablespoons fresh lemon juice
1 clove garlic, minced
1 teaspoon chopped fresh thyme
1 teaspoon Dijon mustard
⅛ teaspoon kosher salt (optional)
2 tablespoons olive oil

1 large bulb fennel or 2 small bulbs, root end trimmed
2 small red new potatoes (about 6 ounces total), cut into 4 slices
2 red bell peppers, seeded, cut into quarters lengthwise
1 sweet onion (such as Vidalia, Walla Walla, Maui, or Texas 1015), cut into ½-inch-thick slices

freshly ground pepper to taste
4 6-inch whole wheat pita breads, halved and opened
2 cups shredded romaine lettuce leaves

In a small cup, whisk together the ingredients for the marinade; set aside.

Cut the stalks off the fennel where they meet the bulb. Cut into ½-inch-thick slices, making sure each has a piece of the root so that it remains intact. Place in a large nonstick skillet and add the potatoes. Cover with water and simmer until the vegetables are tender when tested with the tip of a sharp knife, about 3 minutes. Drain and place on a baking sheet. Place the peppers and onion slices on the same baking sheet.

Brush all the vegetables with some of the marinade on both sides. Allow to marinate 30 minutes.

Meanwhile, light a grill or preheat the broiler.

Grill or broil the vegetables until they brown, about 3 or 4 minutes per side, basting once on each side with the marinade. Remove from the heat. Season with pepper. Allow the vegetables to cool to room temperature or refrigerate.

To make sandwiches, stuff each pita with ½ cup romaine and then with equal amounts of the vegetables.

Makes 4 servings.

JOSLIN CHOICES: 2 carbohydrate (bread/starch), 2 vegetable, I fat
PER SERVING: 305 calories (25% calories from fat), 9 g total fat (I g saturated fat), 9 g
   protein, 5I g carbohydrates, 9 g dietary fiber, 0 cholesterol, 467 mg sodium, 739 mg
   potassium

Lentil Sandwiches with Spinach and Feta

*P*erfect for a picnic or lunch on the terrace, these sandwiches are so delicious and simple to assemble, you will make them often.

1½ cups dried green or brown lentils, rinsed and picked over
1 large onion, halved

2 large cloves garlic, peeled
2 small bay leaves
2 sprigs fresh thyme or ½ teaspoon crushed dried
2½ tablespoons olive oil
2½ tablespoons white wine vinegar
½ teaspoon salt (optional)
freshly ground pepper to taste
6 6-inch whole wheat pita breads, cut into halves
3 large plum tomatoes (about 1 pound total), thinly sliced
1 small red onion, quartered and thinly sliced
1 bunch baby spinach leaves, washed and dried
2 ounces low-fat feta cheese
fresh thyme leaves for garnish

Place the lentils, onion, garlic, bay leaves, and thyme in a nonstick saucepan. Cover with cold water by 1 inch. Place over high heat; bring to a boil. Reduce the heat and simmer, uncovered, for 25 to 30 minutes, until the lentils are tender but not mushy, adding more water as needed. Drain, returning the lentils to the pan and discarding the onion, garlic, bay leaves, and thyme sprigs.

In a small cup, whisk together the olive oil, vinegar, salt (if using), and pepper. Drizzle over the lentil mixture; toss gently. Transfer to a bowl, cover, and chill until ready to serve.

To serve, place ¼ cup of the lentils in each pita half. Stuff the pita with tomato slices, red onion slices, and spinach leaves. Sprinkle some of the feta cheese on top and garnish with thyme leaves.

Makes 6 servings.

JOSLIN CHOICES: 2 low-fat protein, 3 carbohydrate (bread/starch), 1 fat
PER SERVING: 432 calories (19% calories from fat), 10 g total fat (2 g saturated fat), 23 g
protein, 68 g carbohydrates, 21 g dietary fiber, 5 mg cholesterol, 564 mg sodium, 732 mg
potassium

Wild Mushroom and Farmer's Cheese Omelet in Pitas

*E*ggs make delicious fillings for sandwiches, whether served hot for a meal or cold for lunch. Our combination of ingredients changes this from a plain egg sandwich into a gourmet meal. Add seasonal fresh fruit and you have a light supper to remember.

butter-flavored cooking spray
2 shallots, minced
1 3.2-ounce package shiitake mushrooms, cleaned, stems removed, and thinly sliced
1 6-ounce package Italian cremini mushrooms, cleaned and thinly sliced
2 teaspoons fresh thyme leaves, chopped, or ¼ teaspoon crushed dried
1 tablespoon chopped flat-leaf parsley
freshly ground pepper to taste
2 cups egg substitute
4 ounces farmer's cheese, crumbled
4 6-inch whole wheat pita breads

Lightly coat a nonstick skillet with cooking spray. Add the shallots and sauté over low heat until soft, about 3 minutes. Remove from the skillet. Raise the heat to medium-high, coat the skillet again, and add the mushrooms. Cook, stirring occasionally, until soft and all liquid has evaporated, about 5 minutes. Return the shallots to the skillet and add the thyme, parsley, and pepper. Cook over medium heat, stirring constantly, for 1 minute. Remove from the heat and set aside.

Coat a second nonstick skillet with cooking spray. Add half of the egg substitute and half of the cheese. Cook over medium heat without stirring until the omelet starts to bubble around the edges, about 10 seconds. Then stir, pushing the mixture toward the center of the pan.

When the bottom is set but the top is still slightly wet and creamy, carefully place half of the mushroom mixture down the middle and flip one half of the omelet over the other half to enclose the mushrooms, forming a half circle. Flip out onto a plate to cool.

Make a second omelet in the same manner.

To serve, cut each omelet in half. Lightly coat the pita breads with cooking spray. Place the omelet sections on the bread and carefully roll up the pita. Or cut the pita breads in half, stuffing one half inside the other (see page 104), and place the omelet section in the pita. Serve either warm or cooled.

Makes 4 servings.

JOSLIN CHOICES: 3 low-fat protein, 2½ carbohydrate (bread/starch)
PER SERVING: 382 calories (29% calories from fat), 13 g total fat (6 g saturated fat), 27 g
   protein, 43 g carbohydrates, 7 g dietary fiber, 23 mg cholesterol, 694 mg sodium, 604 mg
   potassium

Artichoke and Feta Pizza

*P*izza does not have to include mozzarella and tomato sauce. It can reflect different flavors of the Mediterranean, as this one does. Years ago we were served a similar pizza as an hors d'oeuvre at a wharf-side taverna on Mykonos, one of the more popular of the Greek islands.

1 11½-inch thin-crust Italian bread shell
olive oil cooking spray
2 tablespoons tomato paste
2 teaspoons water
¼ teaspoon garlic powder
¼ cup chopped fresh basil
2 tablespoons chopped fresh Greek oregano
freshly ground pepper to taste
2 roasted red and yellow bell peppers, peeled, seeded, and cut into strips
1 10-ounce package frozen artichoke hearts, thawed and quartered
2 teaspoons fresh lemon juice
3 ounces low-fat feta cheese, crumbled
2 Italian olives, chopped

Place a pizza stone (if using) in the oven and preheat the oven to 450°F.
   Lightly coat the bread shell with cooking spray. Dilute the tomato paste with wa-

ter so that it is easily spread over the shell, leaving a 1-inch border. Sprinkle with the garlic powder, half of the basil, half of the oregano, and pepper.

Arrange strips of roasted bell peppers and quartered artichoke hearts on the shell. Sprinkle with the lemon juice, crumbled feta cheese, olives, and the remaining basil and oregano. Lightly spray the top with cooking spray. Slide onto the preheated pizza stone (or a heavy baking sheet).

Bake for 15 to 18 minutes, until the cheese and vegetables begin to brown. Serve immediately.

Makes 4 servings.

JOSLIN CHOICES: 1 very-low-fat protein, 2 carbohydrate (bread/starch), 1 vegetable, 1 fat
PER SERVING: 292 calories (20% calories from fat), 7 g total fat (3 g saturated fat), 15 g
protein, 45 mg carbohydrates, 9 g dietary fiber, 11 mg cholesterol, 583 mg sodium, 527 mg
potassium

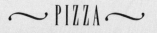

PIZZA

*J*ust about everyone craves this Italian-style dish, but many pizzas are laden with fats that make them difficult to fit into a diabetes meal plan or heart-healthy diet. Here are five pizzas that reflect the trend of combining lower fat ingredients to produce a meal on a crust that needs only a salad to make a complete lunch or dinner.

If you do not have a pizza stone, you may wish to invest in one. They are available in most housewares sections of department stores or in specialty cookware shops. Otherwise, use the heaviest baking sheet you own.

Eggplant and Tomato Pizza

This pizza uses herbed ricotta cheese as a base and melds its tangy flavor with those of eggplant and tomatoes to make a new classic.

olive oil cooking spray
1 small eggplant (about ¾ pound), peeled and sliced into rounds ⅓ inch thick
1 cup low-fat ricotta cheese
2 tablespoons egg substitute
¼ teaspoon garlic powder
⅓ cup chopped fresh basil
½ teaspoon salt (optional)
freshly ground pepper to taste
1 11½-inch thin-crust Italian bread shell
2 large plum tomatoes, thinly sliced
2 tablespoons freshly grated Parmesan cheese

Preheat the broiler. Lightly coat a nonstick baking sheet with cooking spray.

Place the eggplant slices on the prepared pan. Lightly coat the tops of the slices with cooking spray and broil on both sides until browned and tender, about 4 to 5 minutes per side. Set aside.

Place a pizza stone (if using) in the oven and preheat the oven to 450°F.

In a bowl, combine the ricotta, egg substitute, garlic powder, basil, salt (if using), and pepper. Coat the bread shell with cooking spray. Spread with the ricotta cheese mixture, using a spatula to cover the shell but leaving a rim. Top with the cooked eggplant slices and then the tomato slices. Sprinkle with the Parmesan cheese. Slide onto the pizza stone (or a heavy baking sheet). Bake 15 to 20 minutes, until the tomatoes are soft and the cheese has browned. Serve immediately.

Makes 4 servings.

JOSLIN CHOICES: 1 low-fat protein, 2 carbohydrate (bread/starch), 1 vegetable, 1 fat
PER SERVING: 298 calories (25% calories from fat), 8 g total fat (4 g saturated fat), 16 g
    protein, 40 g carbohydrates, 4 g dietary fiber, 21 mg cholesterol, 796 mg sodium, 444 mg
    potassium

Mixed Mushroom Pizza

$\mathcal{D}$ried mushrooms as well as a variety of fresh are available year-round in most markets. The range of tastes and textures is always a pleasant, earthy surprise.

olive oil cooking spray
1 red onion, thinly sliced
½ ounce dried porcini mushrooms, reconstituted according to package directions
½ pound mixed fresh shiitake and cremini mushrooms, thinly sliced
2 cloves garlic, minced
2 tablespoons chopped fresh thyme
½ teaspoon salt (optional)
⅛ teaspoon crushed red pepper flakes
1 11½-inch thin-crust Italian bread shell
1 cup grated skim milk cheddar cheese
2 plum tomatoes, very thinly sliced

Place a pizza stone (if using) in the oven and preheat the oven to 450°F.

Lightly coat a nonstick skillet with cooking spray. Break the onion into rings and sauté until they are soft and caramelized, about 6 minutes. Remove the onion from the skillet and set aside.

Again lightly coat the skillet with cooking spray and sauté the porcini mushrooms for 2 minutes. Add the mixed fresh mushrooms and cook quickly over medium-high heat until the liquid is almost evaporated. Lower the heat and add the garlic. Stir and cook 1 minute longer. Add 1 tablespoon of the thyme, the salt (if using), and the red pepper flakes; set aside.

Coat the bread shell with cooking spray. Sprinkle with ¾ cup cheddar cheese. Top with slices of tomato, the cooked onion rings, and the cooked mushrooms. Sprinkle with the remaining thyme and cheese. Lightly coat the top with cooking spray. Slide the pizza onto the pizza stone (or a heavy baking sheet) and bake for 15 to 18 minutes, until the cheese is melted and the edges are browned. Serve immediately.

Makes 4 servings.

JOSLIN CHOICES: 1 very-low-fat protein, 3 carbohydrate (3 bread/starch)

PER SERVING: 291 calories (14% calories from fat), 5 g total fat (2 g saturated fat), 16 g
protein, 48 g carbohydrates, 4 g dietary fiber, 6 mg cholesterol, 864 mg sodium, 209 mg
potassium

White Pizza

*W*hite pizza is wonderful as an appetizer, cubed to use as a topping for a green mixed salad, or alone as the main course of a meal.

1 11½-inch thin-crust Italian bread shell
olive oil cooking spray
¼ teaspoon garlic powder
1¼ cups shredded nonfat mozzarella cheese
2 tablespoons freshly grated Parmesan cheese
1 tablespoon chopped fresh oregano
1 tablespoon chopped fresh basil
freshly ground pepper to taste

Place a pizza stone (if using) in the oven and preheat the oven to 450°F.

Lightly coat the bread shell with cooking spray. Sprinkle with the garlic powder. Cover with the mozzarella and Parmesan cheese. Sprinkle with the chopped oregano and basil and season with pepper. Lightly coat the top of the pizza with cooking spray and slide onto the pizza stone (or a heavy baking sheet).

Bake for 15 to 18 minutes, until the cheeses are melted and start to brown. Serve immediately.

Makes 4 servings.

JOSLIN CHOICES: 2 very-low-fat protein, 2 carbohydrate (bread/starch)
PER SERVING: 241 calories (12% calories from fat), 3 g total fat (1 g saturated fat), 18 g
protein, 33 g carbohydrates, 2 g dietary fiber, 6 mg cholesterol, 759 mg sodium, 123 mg
potassium

VARIATIONS

- Top the pizza with 2 tablespoons chopped Italian or Greek olives.
- Top the pizza with 1 tablespoon chopped large capers.
- Substitute crumbled low-fat feta cheese for the Parmesan.

Zucchini with Cherry Tomato Pizza

*W*hen cherry tomatoes are heavy on the plants in your garden and zucchini vines are full, it is a good time to make this pizza—sure to please the most discriminating palate. Select the smallest zucchini you can find, as they are the sweetest and have far fewer seeds than larger ones. Substitute small summer squash (yellow or pattypan) for some or all of the zucchini if desired.

olive oil cooking spray
4 small zucchini, sliced into thin rounds
2 cloves garlic, minced
¼ teaspoon salt (optional)
freshly ground pepper to taste
1 11½-inch thin-crust Italian bread shell
½ pound cherry tomatoes, halved
1 cup grated nonfat mozzarella cheese
2 tablespoons freshly grated Parmesan cheese
2 tablespoons chopped fresh basil
1 teaspoon chopped fresh thyme

Place a pizza stone (if using) in the oven and preheat the oven to 450°F.

Lightly coat a nonstick skillet with cooking spray. Add the zucchini and sauté over medium heat until softened and beginning to brown, about 5 minutes. Add the garlic and continue to cook for 1 minute. Season with salt (if using) and pepper. Remove from the heat and set aside.

Lightly coat the bread shell with cooking spray. Place the zucchini on the shell and top with the tomato halves. Cover with the mozzarella and Parmesan cheese. Sprinkle with the basil and thyme. Lightly coat the top of the pizza with cooking spray and slide onto the pizza stone (or a heavy baking sheet). Bake for 15 to 18 minutes, until the tomatoes and cheeses begin to brown. Serve immediately.

Makes 4 servings.

JOSLIN CHOICES: I low-fat protein, 2 carbohydrate (bread/starch), I vegetable
PER SERVING: 264 calories (12% calories from fat), 4 g total fat (I g saturated fat), 18 g
     protein, 40 g carbohydrates, 5 g dietary fiber, 8 mg cholesterol, 809 mg sodium, 693 mg
     potassium

Cheese and Herb Pancakes

*P*ancakes need not be sweet, topped with syrup or fruit. To prove this point, try these light and very tasty little savory pancakes, which are perfect for breakfast, brunch, or lunch.

¾ cup unbleached all-purpose flour
1¼ teaspoons baking powder
⅛ teaspoon salt (optional)
¼ cup egg substitute
¾ cup plus 1 tablespoon skim milk
1 tablespoon chopped fresh basil
½ teaspoon minced fresh thyme
1 teaspoon chopped fresh rosemary
2 tablespoons grated skim milk Swiss cheese
2 tablespoons grated Parmesan cheese
butter-flavored cooking spray
4 tablespoons fat-free sour cream

Combine the flour, baking powder, salt (if using), egg substitute, and milk in a bowl to make a thin pancake batter. Stir in the herbs and grated cheeses.

Coat a nonstick skillet with cooking spray and heat until hot but not smoking. Ladle batter into the skillet, making pancakes about 3 inches in diameter. When the edges brown and the top bubbles, turn over and continue to cook until the bottom is nicely browned, 1 to 2 minutes. Transfer to a plate and keep warm. Repeat, cooking the remaining batter. Top each 2-pancake serving with a tablespoon of the sour cream and serve immediately.

Makes 4 servings, or 8 pancakes.

JOSLIN CHOICES: 1 low-fat protein, 1½ carbohydrate (bread/starch)

PER SERVING: 165 calories (16% calories from fat), 3 g total fat (2 g saturated fat), 10 g
protein, 24 g carbohydrates, 1 g dietary fiber, 9 mg cholesterol, 360 mg sodium, 208 mg
potassium

Country-Style French Toast

*T*his breakfast treat will be a hit with young and old alike. You can pulverize the cereal in a food processor or place it in a self-sealing plastic bag and crush with a rolling pin.

¾ cup egg substitute
⅓ cup skim milk
½ teaspoon ground cinnamon
⅛ teaspoon ground nutmeg
8 1-inch-thick slices French bread
1 cup Special K cereal, reduced to fine crumbs
butter-flavored cooking spray
maple-flavored sugar-free syrup or sugar-free fruit-flavored syrup, warmed

In a shallow dish, whisk together the egg substitute, milk, cinnamon, and nutmeg. Place the bread slices in the egg mixture and turn to coat both sides. Dip the bread slices in cereal crumbs.

Generously coat a cast-iron or heavy nonstick skillet with cooking spray. Place over medium-high heat. Add the coated bread slices to the pan and cook, turning once, until both sides are nicely browned, about 3 to 4 minutes per side.

Transfer the cooked bread slices to a warmed platter and repeat the process until all the bread is cooked. Serve hot with syrup.

Makes 4 servings.

JOSLIN CHOICES: I very-low-fat protein, 2½ carbohydrate (bread/starch)

PER SERVING: 221 calories (13% calories from fat), 3 g total fat (I g saturated fat), 12 g
protein, 36 g carbohydrates, 2 g dietary fiber, I mg cholesterol, 485 mg sodium, 261 mg
potassium

Oatmeal Yogurt Muffins

*W*hen first diagnosed with diabetes, you may think that cakes and muffins will forever be just memories, but these delicious morsels disprove that thought. Although they have healthy ingredients like oatmeal and yogurt, the end result is a muffin with a crisp crust and a soft, fragrant interior. Sunday brunch is back again.

vegetable cooking spray
¾ cup unbleached all-purpose flour
¾ cup rolled oats
2 tablespoons sugar
⅛ teaspoon sugar substitute
1 teaspoon baking powder
½ teaspoon baking soda
1 teaspoon ground cinnamon
½ cup plain nonfat yogurt
⅓ cup skim milk
1½ tablespoons stick margarine, melted
¼ cup egg substitute
2 teaspoons grated orange zest

Preheat the oven to 400°F. Lightly coat 8 ⅓-cup nonstick muffin cups with cooking spray.

In a mixing bowl, combine the flour, oats, sugar, sugar substitute, baking powder, baking soda, and cinnamon. Stir to combine. Add the yogurt, milk, margarine, egg substitute, and orange zest. Mix with a spoon until combined.

Fill each muffin cup ⅔ full. Bake for 25 to 30 minutes, until browned and a tester inserted in the center of a muffin comes out clean. Serve warm.

Makes 8 muffins.

JOSLIN CHOICES: 1 carbohydrate (bread/starch)
PER 1-MUFFIN SERVING: 116 calories (19% calories from fat), 2 g total fat (1 g saturated fat),
    4 g protein, 19 g carbohydrates, 1 g dietary fiber, 1 mg cholesterol, 194 mg sodium, 85 mg
    potassium

Raspberry Yogurt Muffins

*P*erfect for breakfast or brunch, these melt-in-the-mouth muffins are moist and filled with luscious fruit flavor. They're a snap to make and are also delicious with fresh blueberries or blackberries.

> *vegetable cooking spray*
> *2 cups unbleached all-purpose flour*
> *⅓ cup sugar*
> *1 teaspoon baking powder*
> *1 teaspoon baking soda*
> *¼ teaspoon salt*
> *¼ cup fresh orange juice*
> *2 tablespoons canola oil*
> *½ teaspoon almond extract*
> *1 8-ounce container nonfat vanilla yogurt*
> *1 large egg, lightly beaten, or ¼ cup egg substitute*
> *1 cup fresh or frozen raspberries*
> *2 tablespoons sliced almonds*

Preheat the oven to 400°F. Lightly coat 12 muffin cups with cooking spray or line with paper muffin liners.

In a large bowl, combine the flour, sugar, baking powder, baking soda, and salt. Make a well in the center.

In another bowl, whisk together the orange juice, oil, almond extract, yogurt, and egg. Add to the dry ingredients and stir just until the dry ingredients are moistened. Do not overmix. Gently fold in the raspberries.

Divide the batter among the muffin cups and sprinkle each with some of the sliced almonds. Bake until golden, about 16 to 18 minutes. Remove from the pan and let cool on a wire rack.

Makes 12 muffins.

JOSLIN CHOICES: 2 carbohydrate (bread/starch)

PER 1-MUFFIN SERVING: 156 calories (20% calories from fat), 3 g total fat (0 saturated fat),
    4 g protein, 27 g carbohydrates, 1 g dietary fiber, 18 mg cholesterol, 192 mg sodium,
    113 mg potassium

PASTA

Linguine with Asparagus, Fresh Herbs, and Lemon

$\mathcal{E}$ach spring we eagerly await the first crocus and tiny snowdrops in our gardens, as well as reasonably priced fresh asparagus in the supermarket. It's a sign that the worst of winter is almost over and spring is coming fast. At other times of the year, you can substitute broccoli or zucchini for the asparagus.

> 8 ounces dried or fresh linguine
> butter-flavored cooking spray
> 1 tablespoon olive oil
> 1 bunch scallions, white part and 1 inch green, thinly sliced
> 1 pound thin asparagus, tough ends removed, sliced into 1-inch pieces on the
>   diagonal
> 1 tablespoon chopped fresh tarragon or 1 teaspoon crushed dried
> 1 tablespoon chopped walnuts, toasted
> 1 teaspoon grated lemon zest
> 3 tablespoons fresh lemon juice
> 2 tablespoons chopped flat-leaf parsley
> 2 tablespoons grated Parmesan cheese
> freshly ground pepper to taste

Bring a large kettle of lightly salted water to a boil and cook the linguine according to package directions until al dente. Drain and lightly coat with cooking spray.

In a nonstick skillet, heat the olive oil until very hot but not smoking. Add the scallions and asparagus; cook, stirring, until the asparagus is crisp cooked, about 3 minutes. Lower the heat and add the tarragon, toasted walnuts, and reserved linguine. Sprinkle with the lemon zest, lemon juice, and parsley. Toss, then sprinkle with the Parmesan cheese and toss again. Serve at once. Pass the pepper grinder for everyone to add to taste.

Makes 4 servings.

JOSLIN CHOICES: 2 carbohydrate (bread/starch), I vegetable, I fat
PER SERVING: 247 calories (24% calories from fat), 7 g total fat (I g saturated fat), I I g
    protein, 40 g carbohydrates, 5 g dietary fiber, 2 mg cholesterol, 166 mg sodium, 510 mg
    potassium

Fettuccine with Garlic and Broccoli Rabe

This is a great pasta dish. Stronger-flavored than broccoli, broccoli rabe is an Italian delight that's finding its rightful place in American supermarket produce sections. Broccoli may be used in place of the broccoli rabe for a less intense, more straightforward dish.

1 teaspoon olive oil
5 large cloves garlic, thinly sliced
¾ cup canned low-fat, low-sodium chicken or vegetable broth
8 ounces fettuccine
2 bunches broccoli rabe, coarsely chopped
grated zest and juice of 1 lemon
salt to taste (optional)
freshly ground pepper to taste
½ cup freshly grated Parmesan cheese
½ cup chopped flat-leaf parsley
3 tablespoons dry bread crumbs
½ teaspoon crushed red pepper flakes

In a heavy nonstick skillet, heat the oil over medium-low heat. Add the garlic and sauté, stirring occasionally, until golden but not browned, about 5 minutes. Add the broth and bring to a slow simmer.

Meanwhile, cook the fettuccine according to package directions until al dente.

While the pasta is cooking, add the broccoli rabe to the simmering broth. Cook, covered, for 2 to 3 minutes.

Drain the pasta and place in a large pasta bowl. Add the lemon zest and juice. Toss. Pour the broth and broccoli rabe over the pasta; toss again. Season with salt (if using) and pepper. Add the Parmesan cheese, parsley, bread crumbs, and red pepper flakes. Toss well and serve at once.

Makes 4 servings.

JOSLIN CHOICES: 1 low-fat protein, 3 carbohydrate (bread/starch), 1 vegetable
PER SERVING: 339 calories (17% calories from fat), 7 g total fat (3 g saturated fat), 19 g protein, 55 g carbohydrates, 3 g dietary fiber, 11 mg cholesterol, 336 mg sodium, 204 mg potassium

Cooking Pasta

For 1 pound of pasta, use 4 quarts of rapidly boiling water. For smaller amounts, never use less than 3 quarts of water. Pasta should be cooked until it is firm to the bite, al dente. Overcooked pasta becomes heavy and pasty, losing its ability to deliver the flavors of the sauce.

We suggest draining the pasta when you think it still needs a few seconds of cooking time. During the time that you are draining the pasta, transferring it to a serving bowl, and dressing it with the sauce and other ingredients, the pasta will have cooked a little longer and will be just right.

Toss pasta rapidly, using pasta tools, two forks, or a fork and spoon, reaching down to the bottom of the bowl and lifting and swirling the pasta to separate it and evenly coat it with the sauce.

Gnocchi

*G*nocchi (NYOH-kee) are Italian dumplings. They can be made with semolina, farina, potatoes, or with vegetables like spinach. Here we share a recipe that uses both sweet and baking potatoes. If you are not going to cook the gnocchi within a few hours of making them, refrigerate in a single layer to keep them from becoming sticky.

Use the gnocchi in the recipes that follow. Toss the gnocchi with your favorite fresh tomato sauce, or spritz them with butter-flavored cooking spray and toss with a bit of freshly grated Parmesan cheese and chopped fresh chives.

1 russet potato (about ¾ pound), scrubbed
1 sweet potato (about ¾ pound), scrubbed
2 tablespoons egg substitute
¾ cup unbleached all-purpose flour

Boil the potatoes, unpeeled, in lightly salted boiling water until tender when pierced with a fork, about 25 to 30 minutes. Cool slightly and peel. Mash or rice the potatoes (do not puree in a food processor). Stir in the egg substitute and flour. Knead to form a soft dough. If too sticky to handle, add a bit more flour.

Coat your hands with flour. Divide the dough into 4 pieces and roll each into a log about 1½ inches in diameter. Cut the dough into ½-inch-thick slices. Roll the pieces of dough with the tines of a floured fork to score the gnocchi.

Bring a large pot of lightly salted water to a slow boil. Drop the gnocchi into the water, a few at a time. They are done when they rise to the top. Remove with a slotted spoon and drain. Continue until all the gnocchi are cooked.

Makes 4 servings.

JOSLIN CHOICES: 2 carbohydrate (bread/starch)
PER SERVING (Gnocchi only): 160 calories (3% calories from fat), 1 g total fat (0 saturated
fat), 5 g protein, 33 g carbohydrates, 2 g dietary fiber, 0 cholesterol, 19 mg sodium, 377 mg
potassium

Gnocchi with Broccoli, Sicilian-Style

$\mathcal{T}$his is a recipe reminiscent of true southern Italian cooking. Have some low-fat cheese and fresh fruit for dessert. You'll almost be able to smell the wild herbs that cover the countryside of the sunny island of Sicily.

2½ pounds fresh broccoli
olive oil cooking spray
½ medium onion, chopped
2 cloves garlic, minced
2 teaspoons capers, chopped if large
2 teaspoons dried currants
1 recipe gnocchi (page 122), cooked, with ½ cup cooking water reserved

Cut the broccoli into florets and dice the stems into bite-size pieces. Peel the stems if tough. Place the broccoli in a large shallow microwave-safe dish. Cover and microwave on high for 5 to 7 minutes. Drain and set aside.

Lightly coat a nonstick skillet with cooking spray. Add the onion and garlic. Cook, stirring, over medium heat until the onion begins to wilt, about 4 minutes. Add the broccoli, capers, currants, and reserved gnocchi cooking water. Cook over high heat until the water evaporates and the broccoli is crisp cooked.

Place the gnocchi in a microwave-safe casserole. Spoon the broccoli mixture on top and reheat in the microwave for 1 to 2 minutes. Serve immediately.

Makes 4 servings.

JOSLIN CHOICES: 1 very-low-fat protein, 3 carbohydrate (bread/starch)
PER SERVING: 256 calories (5% calories from fat), 2 g total fat (0 saturated fat), 14 g protein,
    52 g carbohydrates, 5 g dietary fiber, 0 cholesterol, 149 mg sodium, 1,277 mg potassium

Gnocchi with Fresh Tomato Mushroom Sauce

*I*n the summer, use fresh tomatoes from the garden for this dish, and in the winter, fresh plum tomatoes. Try different mixes of mushrooms for variation—chanterelles and shiitake, morels, oyster, or porcini—whatever looks good at your supermarket or produce stand.

> *1 tablespoon olive oil*
> *12 ounces mixed cremini and portobello mushrooms, sliced*
> *2 cloves garlic, minced*
> *1½ pounds fresh tomatoes, peeled and chopped*
> *⅛ teaspoon crushed red pepper flakes, or to taste*
> *3 tablespoons chopped flat-leaf parsley*
> *2 tablespoons chopped fresh basil*
> *1 recipe gnocchi (page 122), cooked*
> *2 tablespoons grated Parmesan cheese*

Preheat the oven to 350°F.

Heat the oil in a large nonstick skillet. Add the mushrooms and cook, stirring, until they begin to soften. Add the garlic and cook 1 minute. Stir in the tomatoes and their juices and the red pepper flakes. Raise the heat to high and cook until the sauce thickens. Add the parsley and basil; simmer for 2 minutes.

Place the cooked gnocchi in an ovenproof dish. Pour the tomato sauce over the gnocchi and top with the Parmesan cheese. Bake, uncovered, until the sauce is bubbly and the cheese melts, about 15 to 20 minutes. Serve immediately.

Makes 4 servings.

JOSLIN CHOICES: 2 carbohydrate (bread/starch), 2 vegetable, 1 fat
PER SERVING: 271 calories (18% calories from fat), 6 g total fat (1 g saturated fat), 11 g
protein, 46 g carbohydrates, 6 g dietary fiber, 3 mg cholesterol, 115 mg sodium, 713 mg
potassium

Tomato Tidbits

Nowadays, if you're willing to pay the price, you can buy wonderful tomatoes with exceptional flavor year-round, sometimes still attached to the vine. During the winter they will have been flown in by overnight jet freight from Australia, South or Central America, or Israel. Handle these beauties correctly and you have the full flavor of just-picked tomatoes whenever you want.

The main rule for tomatoes: NEVER store a tomato in the refrigerator and never buy a tomato from a refrigerated case. Temperatures below 55°F will destroy the flavor and aroma of the tomato, as well as the tomato's ability to keep ripening. Always store tomatoes at room temperature.

Next, if you're buying tomatoes in advance of their use, pick firm, well-colored tomatoes that are not yet soft and ripe. Use them as they ripen and yield gently to pressure. They'll ripen sooner in a sunny windowsill. To hold them longer, keep them in a dark, well-ventilated place that's out of direct sunlight.

Lastly, cut a tomato just before you intend to serve it. Tomatoes will lose their aroma within 15 minutes of cutting, so no slicing hours ahead. If adding a dressing to tomatoes, use just a drizzle so the wonderful flavor of the tomato is not overpowered.

Rigatoni with Lemon-Parsley Pesto

Parsley and lemon make a bright-flavored pesto when your garden basil is done and the store variety is too expensive.

> 12 ounces rigatoni or other tubular-shaped pasta
> 1 lemon
> 2 cups tightly packed flat-leaf parsley leaves
> 2 ounces freshly grated Parmesan cheese
> 2 tablespoons olive oil

In a large pot of water, cook the rigatoni according to package directions until al dente.

Meanwhile, using a vegetable peeler, pare the zest of the lemon into long, thin strips. Set a few strips aside for garnish. Place the remaining lemon zest, 2 tablespoons lemon juice, parsley, and Parmesan cheese in a food processor fitted with a metal blade. Process until the parsley is finely minced. With the motor running, drizzle the olive oil through the feed tube and pulse until the pesto is smooth, scraping down the sides of the work bowl occasionally.

When the pasta is done, drain and place in a large bowl. Spoon the pesto over the pasta and toss to coat evenly. Serve at once.

Makes 6 servings.

JOSLIN CHOICES: 3 carbohydrate (bread/starch), 1 fat
PER SERVING: 295 calories (26% calories from fat), 9 g total fat (3 g saturated fat), 12 g
    protein, 44 g carbohydrates, 2 g dietary fiber, 7 mg cholesterol, 187 mg sodium, 234 mg
    potassium

Mango and Pasta Salad

We love mangoes, and happily, our supermarket frequently sells them at three (sometimes five during peak seasons) for a dollar. Once you've mastered how to cut a mango (page 56), you'll find yourself adding its exotic flavor—frequently described as a combination of pineapple, peach, and apricot—to all kinds of dishes.

Here we've teamed mango with farfalle (bow-tie) pasta for a flavor-packed pasta dish that can be served as a main course or as a side dish in a more elaborate meal.

> *4 quarts water*
> *12 ounces farfalle (bow-tie pasta) or other whimsical dried pasta shape*
> *1 large ripe mango*
> *⅓ cup minced fresh cilantro*
> *2 tablespoons fresh lime juice*
> *2 tablespoons seasoned rice vinegar*
> *1 teaspoon finely grated fresh ginger*

½ teaspoon dark sesame oil
freshly ground pepper to taste

In a large pot, bring the water to a rapid boil. Add the pasta and cook just until al dente, about 7 to 9 minutes, or cook according to package directions. Drain the pasta and place in a large shallow pasta bowl or on a large platter.

Peel and thinly slice the mango. Scatter the mango pieces and cilantro over the pasta. In a small cup, whisk together the lime juice, vinegar, ginger, and sesame oil. Drizzle over the pasta and lightly toss. Season with pepper and serve warm or at room temperature.

Makes 6 servings.

JOSLIN CHOICES: 3 carbohydrate (bread/starch)
PER SERVING: 223 calories (6% calories from fat), 1 g total fat (0 saturated fat), 7 g protein, 46 g carbohydrates, 2 g dietary fiber, 0 cholesterol, 2 mg sodium, 108 mg potassium

Dried and Fresh Mushrooms with Linguine

*I*n Italy and in large American cities, both fresh and dried porcini mushrooms are available in stores, but in many sections of the country, we are forced to buy a combination of dried Italian mushrooms. No matter what is available to you, this dish is always a marvel of flavors.

¾ ounce dried Italian mushrooms
8 ounces linguine
½ tablespoon olive oil
6 ounces cremini mushrooms, quartered
3 cloves garlic, thinly sliced
¼ cup dry white wine or fresh lemon juice
⅓ cup canned low-fat, low-sodium chicken broth or pasta cooking water
¼ cup chopped flat-leaf parsley
⅛ teaspoon crushed red pepper flakes
2 tablespoons grated Parmesan cheese

Rehydrate the dried mushrooms according to package directions. Drain and set aside.

Bring a large kettle of water to a boil and cook the pasta according to package directions until al dente.

Heat the oil in a large nonstick skillet until very hot but not smoking. Add the reconstituted and fresh mushrooms and garlic; cook, stirring, for 1 minute. Add the wine and continue to cook and stir for another minute. Stir in the broth or pasta water. Cook until the mushrooms are tender, about 6 to 8 minutes. Turn down the heat and add the parsley and red pepper flakes.

Drain the cooked pasta and toss with the mushroom sauce. Sprinkle with the Parmesan cheese and serve immediately.

Makes 4 servings.

JOSLIN CHOICES: 1 low-fat protein, 1 carbohydrate (bread/starch)
PER SERVING: 160 calories (19% calories from fat), 3 g total fat (1 g saturated fat), 8 g
     protein, 21 g carbohydrates, 3 g dietary fiber, 3 mg cholesterol, 89 mg sodium, 63 mg
     potassium

Sautéed Okra and Tomatoes over Pasta

*W*e love okra in just about any form, but this rustic combination of fresh okra, onions, and plum tomatoes makes a terrific topping for pasta. The last-minute addition of lemon juice gives this peasant dish a bright tang.

When buying okra, look for small buds, 3 to 4 inches long, that are an even green color. Be careful when trimming the ends not to cut into the pod—just slice off the stem end.

> *olive oil cooking spray*
> *1 tablespoon olive oil*
> *1 medium onion, finely chopped*
> *2 large cloves garlic, minced*
> *1 pound small green okra, stem ends trimmed*
> *½ pound ripe plum tomatoes, cored and coarsely chopped*
> *salt to taste (optional)*

freshly ground pepper to taste
12 ounces rotelle (corkscrew pasta)
1 tablespoon fresh lemon juice
¼ teaspoon crushed red pepper flakes, or to taste

Lightly coat a large nonstick skillet with cooking spray. Add the olive oil and place over medium heat. Add the onion and garlic; sauté until the onion is limp, stirring occasionally, about 4 minutes. Add the okra and continue to cook, stirring occasionally, until it softens slightly and turns a bright green, about 5 minutes. Stir in the tomatoes and season with salt (if using) and pepper. Simmer over low heat for about 10 minutes.

Meanwhile, in a large pot of boiling water, cook the pasta according to package directions for al dente. Drain.

Place the cooked pasta on a large serving platter or in a pasta bowl. Top with the okra-tomato mixture and drizzle with the lemon juice. Toss. Sprinkle with the red pepper flakes. Serve hot.

Makes 6 servings.

JOSLIN CHOICES: 3 carbohydrate (bread/starch)
PER SERVING: 265 calories (12% calories from fat), 4 g total fat (1 g saturated fat), 10 g protein, 51 g carbohydrates, 5 g dietary fiber, 0 cholesterol, 13 mg sodium, 457 mg potassium

Cold Rice Noodle Salad with Peanut Dressing

*P*eanut oil makes the dressing on this salad highly aromatic. Store the oil in the refrigerator after it has been opened.

12 ounces cellophane rice noodles
2 medium cucumbers, peeled
2 medium carrots, peeled

DRESSING

2 tablespoons roasted peanut oil

1 tablespoon reduced low-sodium soy sauce

juice of 3 fresh limes

1 clove garlic, minced

1 teaspoon minced fresh ginger

2 tablespoons chopped fresh basil

1 tablespoon minced fresh mint

2 tablespoons chopped dry-roasted peanuts for garnish (optional)

Cook the rice noodles according to package directions. Drain and set aside.

Cut the cucumbers in half lengthwise and, using a small spoon, scrape out and discard the seeds. Cut the cucumbers into thin julienne strips about 2 inches long. Cut the carrots into thin julienne strips about 2 inches long. Combine the vegetables and noodles; place in a shallow pasta bowl or on a large platter.

To make the dressing, in a small bowl, whisk together the peanut oil, soy sauce, lime juice, garlic, ginger, basil, and mint. Pour over the noodle mixture and toss to coat evenly. Chill for at least 1 hour or up to 6 hours.

When ready to serve, toss again. Scatter the peanuts (if using) over the top. Serve cold.

Makes 6 servings.

JOSLIN CHOICES: 3 carbohydrate (bread/starch), 1 vegetable, 1 fat
PER SERVING: 295 calories (20% calories from fat), 7 g total fat (1 g saturated fat), 4 g protein,
55 g carbohydrates, 3 g dietary fiber, 0 cholesterol, 205 mg sodium, 282 mg potassium

Pumpkin Ravioli with Mushroom Ragout

Ravioli filled with a velvety pumpkin mousse and topped with a savory ragout of wild mushrooms will become a specialty of your kitchen once you've tasted this delicious rustic pasta dish. Fresh wonton skins are increasingly available at supermarkets and make fine ravioli with little effort.

RAVIOLI

4 shallots, minced, or ¼ cup minced red onion
1 tablespoon olive oil
1 cup fresh or canned pumpkin puree
2 large eggs at room temperature, lightly beaten
½ cup dry unseasoned bread crumbs
¼ cup freshly grated Parmesan cheese
2 tablespoons minced fresh basil
salt to taste (optional)
freshly ground pepper to taste
30 wonton skins

RAGOUT

1 tablespoon stick margarine
1 tablespoon olive oil
1 small onion, finely chopped
1 pound portobello mushrooms, halved if large, thinly sliced
½ pound button mushrooms, thinly sliced
2 cloves garlic, minced
1 teaspoon minced fresh sage or ¼ teaspoon crushed dried
salt to taste (optional)
freshly ground pepper to taste
1 28-ounce can no-salt-added tomatoes with juice, coarsely chopped

To make the ravioli, in a small saucepan, sauté the shallots in the oil over low heat until limp and lightly golden, about 5 minutes. Add the pumpkin puree and simmer about 4 minutes, stirring constantly to prevent scorching. Remove from the heat and whisk in the eggs, bread crumbs, Parmesan cheese, and basil. Taste and season with salt (if using) and pepper.

Put a wonton skin on a lightly floured work surface. Mound 1 level tablespoon of the pumpkin mixture in the center. Brush the edges of the wonton skin with water and fold in half to form a triangle, pressing around the filling with the tines of a fork to force out the air. Transfer the ravioli to a dry kitchen towel. Repeat, making the remaining ravioli.

Meanwhile, to make the mushroom ragout, in a large heavy saucepan, heat the margarine and oil over medium heat until the margarine is melted. Add the onion and cook, stirring, for 4 to 5 minutes, until softened. Stir in all the mushrooms, garlic, sage, salt (if using), and several grinds of pepper. Cook until the liquid that the mushrooms give off is evaporated, about 8 minutes. Stir in the tomatoes and their juice and cook, uncovered, stirring occasionally, until the ragout is thick, about 30 minutes.

When the ragout is almost done, bring a large pot of water to a boil. Add the ravioli and cook until they rise to the surface. Turn over and continue to cook for another 1 to 2 minutes, until tender. Remove the cooked ravioli with a slotted spoon and drain well.

To serve, divide the ravioli among 6 serving plates and top with the ragout. Serve at once.

Makes 6 servings.

JOSLIN CHOICES: 2 carbohydrate (bread/starch), 2 vegetable, 2 fat
PER SERVING: 323 calories (29% calories from fat), 11 g total fat (2 g saturated fat), 14 g
    protein, 46 g carbohydrates, 7 g dietary fiber, 78 mg cholesterol, 44 mg sodium, 61 mg
    potassium

Lo Mein Salad

*W*e've always been intrigued by the amazing range of flavors and textures one can get by using Asian cooking techniques and ingredients to create interesting salads and light main courses. Fortunately, many Asian ingredients are now available at well-stocked supermarkets and Asian grocers throughout the country. Here we've teamed lo mein noodles (you may substitute medium no-egg noodles or linguine) with crisply cooked vegetables and some Asian seasonings, with delicious results.

12 ounces lo mein or medium egg noodles
1 teaspoon dark sesame oil
1 tablespoon canola oil
1 medium onion, cut in half, then thinly sliced
2 large cloves garlic, finely chopped

1 cup broccoli florets
1 cup cauliflower florets
1 medium carrot, halved crosswise, and cut into thin julienne strips
¼ pound snow peas, strings removed
1 cup canned low-fat, low-sodium chicken or vegetable broth
1 tablespoon dry sherry
1 tablespoon reduced-sodium soy sauce
1 tablespoon imported Indian curry powder
¼ to ½ teaspoon crushed red pepper flakes, to taste (optional)
freshly ground pepper to taste

In a large pot, cook the noodles in boiling water until al dente, about 4 to 6 minutes. Drain and place in a large bowl. Drizzle with the sesame oil and toss to coat evenly. Set aside.

Set a wok or large nonstick skillet over high heat and heat the canola oil. Add the onion and garlic, reduce the heat to medium-low, stir-fry until the onion and garlic are limp but not browned. Add the broccoli, cauliflower, and carrot. Stir-fry for 1 minute. Add the snow peas and continue to stir-fry for another 30 seconds.

In a cup, whisk together the broth, sherry, soy sauce, curry powder, and red pepper flakes (if using). Pour into the wok and cook, stirring frequently, until the vegetables are barely tender, 2 to 3 minutes. Add the noodles to the wok and gently toss to mix.

Transfer the noodles and vegetables to a large platter and top with several grinds of pepper. Serve warm or at room temperature.

Makes 6 servings.

JOSLIN CHOICES: 2 carbohydrate (bread/starch), 1 vegetable, 1 fat
PER SERVING: 253 calories (20% calories from fat), 6 g total fat (1 g saturated fat), 9 g
    protein, 42 g carbohydrate, 4 g dietary fiber, 46 mg cholesterol, 131 mg sodium, 260 mg
    potassium

Pasta Primavera with Sun-Dried Tomatoes

*T*his pasta dish is loaded with wonderful fresh veggies that can vary according to what looks best in the market. Once frozen, the sun-dried tomatoes crumble easily with your fingers or a rolling pin. They are also great sprinkled on soups or salads.

8 ounces linguine
4 cups broccoli florets
¼ pound fresh green beans, trimmed and cut into 1-inch pieces
¼ pound fresh asparagus, woody ends removed
¼ pound fresh sugar snap peas, strings removed
4 scallions, white part only, minced
¼ cup chopped fresh dill
1 teaspoon olive oil
2 ounces part-skim mozzarella cheese, shredded
1 ounce dry-packed sun-dried tomatoes, placed in freezer for 5 minutes

Cook the linguine according to package directions until al dente.

Meanwhile, cook the broccoli and green beans in a pot of water to cover until crisp-tender, about 5 minutes. Using a slotted spoon, remove the broccoli and beans. Set aside. Add the asparagus and sugar snap peas to the pot and cook for 3 to 4 minutes. Drain, reserving the cooking liquid.

When the pasta is done, drain and place in a large pasta bowl. Add the broccoli, beans, asparagus, and sugar snap peas. Sprinkle with the scallions and dill. Drizzle with the oil and ⅓ cup of the reserved cooking liquid. Toss. If the pasta seems too dry, drizzle with more reserved cooking liquid and toss again. Sprinkle with the cheese and crumble the sun-dried tomatoes over the top. Serve at once.

Makes 4 servings.

JOSLIN CHOICES: 1 low-fat protein, 2 carbohydrate (bread/starch), 1 vegetable
PER SERVING: 260 calories (17% calories from fat), 5 g total fat (2 g saturated fat), 14 g
protein, 44 g carbohydrates, 7 g dietary fiber, 8 mg cholesterol, 341 mg sodium, 779 mg
potassium

Rotelle Pasta with Swiss Chard, Sage, and Rosemary

*T*his hearty pasta dish combines Italian favorites—pasta and a strong-flavored green—with assertive fresh herbs such as sage and rosemary. If you like, you can substitute another dense pasta, such as penne or ziti, for the rotelle.

8 ounces rotelle (corkscrew pasta)
2 tablespoons olive oil
3 large cloves garlic, minced
1 tablespoon minced fresh sage
2 teaspoons minced fresh rosemary
1 pound Swiss chard, washed and tough stems removed
freshly ground pepper to taste
2 tablespoons grated Parmesan cheese

Cook the pasta according to package directions until al dente.

Meanwhile, heat the oil in a large nonstick skillet over medium-low heat. Sauté the garlic for 2 minutes, until it turns golden. Add the herbs and sauté another minute. Cut the Swiss chard into thin chiffonnade strips and stir into the garlic-herb mixture. Continue to cook until the chard wilts, about 3 minutes.

Remove ¼ cup of the pasta cooking liquid and stir into the skillet. Continue to cook until the pasta is done. Drain the pasta and toss with the chard mixture in the skillet. Sprinkle liberally with pepper. Toss with the cheese and serve immediately.

Makes 4 servings.

JOSLIN CHOICES: 3 carbohydrate (bread/starch), 1 fat
PER SERVING: 307 calories (27% calories from fat), 10 g total fat (2 g saturated fat), 11 g
    protein, 47 g carbohydrates, 4 g dietary fiber, 2 mg cholesterol, 304 mg sodium, 554 mg
    potassium

Thai Noodles with Tofu and Peanuts

Thai food has a wonderful fresh taste, with sauces that do not overwhelm unless you make the mistake of asking for your dinner very spicy. At that point you may need your own fire extinguisher. We love Thai noodles and hope that you will take the time to make this rendition of *pad Thai*.

3½ ounces rice stick noodles
vegetable cooking spray
¾ cup egg substitute
6 ounces firm tofu, pressed, cut into 1 x ½-inch strips (see page 179)
½ teaspoon dark sesame oil
1 bunch scallions, white part and 1 inch green, chopped
2 tablespoons minced fresh garlic
1 to 2 fresh small red chile peppers, seeded and minced (optional)
3 tablespoons Thai fish sauce
¼ cup fresh lemon juice
1½ packets sugar substitute
¼ cup chopped dry-roasted unsalted peanuts
¼ cup chopped fresh basil
⅓ cup fresh cilantro leaves
½ teaspoon crushed red pepper flakes
¼ pound fresh bean sprouts, roots pinched off
lime wedges and cucumber slices for garnish (optional)

Place the rice sticks in a bowl and cover with hot water. Soak for 20 minutes. Drain and cut into 2-inch pieces. Set aside.

Lightly coat a nonstick skillet with cooking spray. Place over medium-low heat, add the egg substitute, and scramble until the eggs are softly set. Set aside.

Coat the tofu with the sesame oil.

Lightly coat a large nonstick skillet with cooking spray. Heat until very hot but not smoking. Stir-fry the scallions, garlic, red chiles, and tofu for 1 minute. Lower the heat and add the fish sauce, lemon juice, and sugar substitute. Add the peanuts, basil, cilantro, and red pepper flakes. Heat through.

Place the noodles on a large serving plate. Top with the tofu mixture and the bean sprouts. If using, garnish with lime wedges and cucumber slices. Serve immediately.

Makes 4 servings.

JOSLIN CHOICES: I medium-fat protein, 2 carbohydrate (bread/starch), I fat
PER SERVING: 278 calories (28% calories from fat), 9 g total fat (I g saturated fat), 15 g protein, 36 g carbohydrates, 3 g dietary fiber, 0 cholesterol, 124 mg sodium, 540 mg potassium

Penne Arrabbiata

This is our favorite version of this pasta dish. With practice you can have the dish ready in 20 minutes, making it perfect for spontaneous midweek entertaining. While you make the pasta, warm some crusty bread and have your guests make the salad. Dessert can be a crisp pear served with a small wedge of low-fat cheese.

8 ounces penne
½ teaspoon crushed red pepper flakes
2 large cloves garlic, finely chopped
1 tablespoon olive oil
1 14½-ounce can no-salt-added whole Italian tomatoes with their juice
2 tablespoons chopped flat-leaf parsley
3 tablespoons freshly grated Parmesan cheese
freshly ground pepper to taste

Cook the pasta according to package directions until al dente.

Meanwhile, in a heavy nonstick skillet, cook the red pepper flakes and garlic in the olive oil over low heat until the pepper flakes are fragrant and the garlic is limp but not browned, about 2 minutes. Add the tomatoes and their juice, breaking up the tomatoes with the back of a wooden spoon. Cook the sauce over medium-low heat until thickened, about 15 minutes.

When the pasta is done, drain and add to the sauce along with the parsley and Parmesan cheese. Toss to coat evenly and serve at once. Pass the pepper grinder.

Makes 4 servings.

JOSLIN CHOICES: I carbohydrate (bread/starch), I vegetable, I fat
PER SERVING: 155 calories (31% calories from fat), 5 g total fat (1 g saturated fat), 6 g
    protein, 22 g carbohydrates, 2 g dietary fiber, 4 mg cholesterol, 99 mg sodium, 281 mg
    potassium

Angel Hair with Tomatoes, Basil, Garlic, Goat Cheese, and Walnuts

This lovely pasta dish relies on very fresh ripe tomatoes and lots of fresh basil and garlic. We spend extra money on the tomatoes, buying those that are sold still attached to the stem. As the ads and billboards say, the tomatoes are "still alive" when they arrive at the store—and your home. They do taste like freshly picked tomatoes.

¼ cup thinly sliced fresh garlic
2 tablespoons olive oil
1 pound very fresh ripe tomatoes, seeded and diced
⅔ cup loosely packed fresh basil leaves, chopped
¾ teaspoon kosher salt (optional)
freshly ground pepper to taste
6 ounces dried or fresh angel hair pasta
2 ounces low-fat goat cheese, crumbled
1 tablespoon chopped walnuts
6 sprigs basil for garnish (optional)

In a heavy skillet over medium-low heat, sauté the garlic slices in olive oil until lightly browned, about 5 minutes. Add the tomatoes, basil, salt (if using), and pepper. Cook for 1 to 2 minutes more, until the tomatoes are just heated through. Remove from the heat, cover, and keep warm.

    Meanwhile, cook the pasta according to package directions until al dente. Drain and transfer to a large shallow pasta bowl or serving platter. Spoon the tomato mixture over the top and sprinkle with the goat cheese and walnuts. Serve at once, tossing the pasta to coat with the other ingredients as you serve in small pasta bowls or on individual plates. If desired, garnish each serving with a sprig of basil. Serve at once.

Makes 6 servings.

JOSLIN CHOICES: 1½ carbohydrate (bread/starch), 2 fat
PER SERVING: 189 calories (41% calories from fat), 9 g total fat (3 g saturated fat), 7 g protein, 22 g carbohydrates, 2 g dietary fiber, 7 mg cholesterol, 388 mg sodium, 290 mg potassium

Stuffed Pasta with Tomato Mushroom Sauce

*F*or this homey casserole, you can use jumbo shells or manicotti tubes. The pasta is filled with a savory stuffing with just the right balance of herbs and cheese, then smothered in a rich vegetable sauce.

12 large pasta shells or manicotti tubes
1 tablespoon olive oil
1 medium onion, minced
2 large cloves garlic, minced
1 cup low-fat ricotta cheese
1 10-ounce package frozen chopped spinach, thawed and squeezed dry
¼ cup freshly grated Romano cheese
2 teaspoons crushed dried oregano
¼ teaspoon freshly ground pepper
⅛ teaspoon ground nutmeg

TOMATO MUSHROOM SAUCE
1 teaspoon olive oil
1 medium onion, chopped
3 large cloves garlic, minced
1 medium red bell pepper, seeded and chopped
½ pound fresh mushrooms, thinly sliced

1 teaspoon crushed dried oregano
1 teaspoon crushed dried basil
1 15-ounce can no-salt-added tomato sauce
1 6-ounce can tomato paste
½ cup dry red wine or water
½ cup shredded part-skim mozzarella cheese

Cook pasta in a large pot of boiling water according to package directions. Drain and set aside.

In a large nonstick skillet, heat the olive oil over medium-low heat. Add the onion and garlic. Sauté, stirring occasionally, until the onion is limp. Remove from the heat. Place the onion mixture in a bowl along with the ricotta cheese, spinach, Romano cheese, oregano, pepper, and nutmeg. Stir to mix well. Use the cheese mixture to lightly stuff the pasta.

To make the sauce, add the olive oil to the same nonstick skillet. Place over medium heat and add the onion, garlic, bell pepper, and mushrooms. Sauté, stirring occasionally, until the vegetables are soft and most of the liquid is evaporated, about 7 minutes. Stir in the oregano, basil, tomato sauce, tomato paste, and wine. Cook, stirring occasionally, until the sauce comes to a boil and thickens slightly.

Spread a fourth of the sauce mixture in a 13 x 9-inch casserole. Top with the filled pasta shells. Spoon the remaining sauce over and around the shells. Sprinkle with the mozzarella cheese. Cover with aluminum foil. (At this point, you may refrigerate for several hours or overnight.)

When ready to bake, preheat the oven to 375°F.

Bake for about 45 to 50 minutes, until heated through and bubbling around the edges. Uncover during the last 15 minutes of baking time to lightly brown the top. Let stand for 5 minutes before serving.

Makes 6 servings.

JOSLIN CHOICES: I low-fat protein, 2 carbohydrate (bread/starch), I fat
PER SERVING: 298 calories (28% calories from fat), 10 g total fat (4 g saturated fat), 16 g

protein, 36 g carbohydrates, 6 g dietary fiber, 22 mg cholesterol, 211 mg sodium, 801 mg

potassium

Vegetable Pastitsio

*T*his casserole of pasta and vegetables brings back fond memories of a seaside taverna on the island of Corfu, where we first sampled this fine example of Greek home cooking. We've taken liberties with the traditional recipe to adapt it to today's lower-fat style of eating.

butter-flavored cooking spray
8 ounces ziti or elbow macaroni
½ cup egg substitute
½ teaspoon salt (optional)
¼ teaspoon ground nutmeg
2 small zucchini, ends trimmed
1 tablespoon reduced-fat margarine
1 small onion, chopped
2 large cloves garlic, minced
1 14½-ounce can no-salt-added crushed tomatoes
1 tablespoon tomato paste
1 cup fresh or frozen corn kernels
½ teaspoon crushed dried oregano
¼ teaspoon crushed dried mint
¼ teaspoon ground cinnamon
¼ teaspoon freshly ground pepper
3 tablespoons unbleached all-purpose flour
½ cup skim milk
¼ cup freshly grated Parmesan cheese

Preheat the oven to 350°F. Lightly coat a 2-quart square casserole with cooking spray.

Cook the pasta according to package directions until al dente. Drain, reserving the cooking liquid. Rinse the pasta with cold water; drain. Place the pasta in a bowl and stir in the egg substitute, ¼ teaspoon salt (if using), and ⅛ teaspoon of the nutmeg. Spread the mixture evenly in the prepared dish. Thinly slice the zucchini lengthwise and arrange over the pasta.

In a nonstick skillet, melt ½ tablespoon margarine over medium-low heat. Add the onion and garlic. Sauté, stirring occasionally, until the onion is limp, about 4 minutes. Add the tomatoes, tomato paste, corn, oregano, mint, cinnamon, pepper, remaining ⅛ teaspoon nutmeg, and remaining ¼ teaspoon salt (if using). Stir until heated through. Spoon the tomato mixture over the zucchini.

In a small saucepan, melt the remaining ½ tablespoon margarine. Stir in the flour and cook for 1 minute. Gradually stir in the milk and cook, stirring, until thick and bubbly, about 3 minutes. Stir in the Parmesan cheese and cook for 1 minute. Spoon the mixture over the top of the casserole.

Bake, uncovered, for 35 to 40 minutes, until the top is firm. Remove from the oven and let stand for 5 minutes before cutting into squares.

Makes 6 servings.

JOSLIN CHOICES: 3 carbohydrate (bread/starch)

PER SERVING: 253 calories (15% calories from fat), 5 g total fat (1 g saturated fat), 12 g
protein, 43 g carbohydrates, 3 g dietary fiber, 4 mg cholesterol, 180 mg sodium, 488 mg
potassium

Grains

Barley Risotto with Portobello Mushrooms

*P*earl barley makes a great substitute for Arborio or Carnaroli (Italian short-grain) rice when making a luscious, creamy risotto. We can buy already cleaned and sliced fresh portobello mushrooms in most supermarkets, which are easy to use and add a "meaty" flavor to the dish.

> *olive oil cooking spray*
> *1 tablespoon olive oil*
> *½ pound sliced fresh portobello mushrooms, cut into 1-inch pieces*
> *1 medium onion, chopped*
> *1 clove garlic, minced*
> *1 cup pearl barley, rinsed*
> *1 tablespoon chopped fresh rosemary or 1 teaspoon crushed dried*
> *¾ cup dry white wine*
> *4 cups canned low-fat, low-sodium chicken or vegetable broth*
> *1 tablespoon slivered blanched almonds, toasted*
> *2 tablespoons chopped flat-leaf parsley*

Lightly coat a large heavy saucepan with cooking spray. Add the olive oil and heat over medium-high heat. Add the mushrooms and cook for 5 to 7 minutes, stirring frequently. Remove the mushrooms and set aside.

Again lightly coat the saucepan with cooking spray. Add the onion and garlic. Cook, stirring often, until the onion wilts, about 4 minutes. Stir in the barley, rosemary, and white wine. Continue to cook for 8 to 10 minutes, stirring often.

Meanwhile, in another saucepan, heat the broth. Add the broth, ½ cup at a time, to the barley, keeping the remaining broth at a slow simmer. Stir the barley mixture frequently, and cook until almost all of the broth has been absorbed before adding the next ½ cup. When the barley is tender and all the broth has been added, stir in the reserved mushrooms. The entire cooking time should take about 35 to 40 minutes. Continue to cook for another 2 to 3 minutes, until the mushrooms are heated through and the risotto reaches the desired consistency. Fold in the almonds and parsley. Serve at once.

Makes 4 servings.

JOSLIN CHOICES: 2 carbohydrate (bread/starch), I vegetable, I fat
PER SERVING: 303 calories (18% calories from fat), 7 g total fat (I g saturated fat), I I g
    protein, 47 g carbohydrates, I I g dietary fiber, 4 mg cholesterol, 391 mg sodium, 253 mg
    potassium

Curried Couscous with Walnuts

*C*ouscous is a staple ingredient in North Africa. Made of semolina, it is quick and easy to prepare and makes a wonderful breakfast cereal, lunch salad, or as in this recipe, dinner side dish.

> *olive oil cooking spray*
> *1 small onion, chopped*
> *2 cloves garlic, minced*
> *¾ to 1 teaspoon curry powder, to taste*
> *1 small red bell pepper, seeded and finely chopped*
> *1½ cups canned low-fat, low-sodium chicken or vegetable broth or water*
> *1½ teaspoons grated lemon zest*
> *2 tablespoons chopped dried apricots*
> *1 cup quick-cooking couscous*
> *⅓ cup chopped fresh mint*
> *1 tablespoon walnut pieces, toasted, for garnish (optional)*

Coat a nonstick skillet with cooking spray. Sauté the onion, garlic, and curry powder for 2 minutes over medium heat until the onion begins to soften. Add the bell pepper and sauté another 3 minutes. Keep warm.

In a covered nonstick pot, bring the broth or water to a boil. Stir in the lemon zest, apricots, and couscous. Cover and remove from the heat. Allow to stand for 5 minutes. Fluff with a fork and stir in the reserved vegetables and mint. If desired, garnish with the toasted walnuts. Serve immediately.

Makes 4 servings.

JOSLIN CHOICES: 2 carbohydrate (bread/starch), 1 vegetable
PER SERVING: 238 calories (9% calories from fat), 2 g total fat (0 saturated fat), 9 g protein,
    45 g carbohydrates, 5 g dietary fiber, 1 mg cholesterol, 66 mg sodium, 238 mg potassium

Couscous with Three Vegetables

*T*his recipe is a meal in one. Dinner can be ready in minutes but tastes as though you've worked for hours at the stove.

   olive oil cooking spray
   1 small onion, chopped
   1 teaspoon turmeric
   1 teaspoon ground cinnamon
   ½ teaspoon chili powder
   1 medium carrot, sliced into thin rounds
   ½ head cauliflower, cut into small florets
   2 medium zucchini, cut into thin rounds
   1½ cups plus 2 tablespoons water or canned low-fat, low-sodium chicken or vegetable
      broth
   2 tablespoons chopped fresh cilantro
   2 tablespoons chopped flat-leaf parsley
   ¼ teaspoon salt (optional)
   1 cup quick-cooking couscous

Lightly coat a nonstick skillet with cooking spray. Sauté the onion for 2 minutes, until softened. Add the turmeric, cinnamon, and chili powder. Cook, stirring, until the spices become fragrant. Add the carrot, cauliflower, zucchini, and 2 tablespoons water or broth. Reduce the heat, cover, and cook until the vegetables are crisp-tender, about 4 to 5 minutes. Stir in the cilantro and parsley. Keep warm.

Bring the remaining 1½ cups water or broth and the salt (if using) to a boil. Stir in the couscous, cover, and remove from the heat. Allow to sit for 5 minutes. Fluff with a fork and stir in the vegetables. Serve immediately.

Makes 4 servings.

JOSLIN CHOICES: 2 carbohydrate (bread/starch), 2 vegetable
PER SERVING: 225 calories (5% calories from fat), 1 g total fat (0 saturated fat), 10 g protein, 45 g carbohydrates, 6 g dietary fiber, 2 mg cholesterol, 223 mg sodium, 604 mg potassium

Kasha with Mushrooms, Peppers, and Bow-Ties

*K*asha (buckwheat groats) and bow-ties is a staple of eastern European dinners, often served as a side dish. Here we add vegetables and a bit of yogurt to make it a meal fit for a czar. For us, this is comfort food from generations gone by.

butter-flavored cooking spray
1 small onion, chopped
4 ounces button mushrooms, sliced
1 red bell pepper, seeded and cut into thin julienne strips
1 cup whole kasha (buckwheat groats)
2 cups canned low-fat, low-sodium chicken broth or mushroom broth
4 ounces bow-tie pasta (farfelle)
freshly ground pepper to taste
¼ cup plain nonfat yogurt, drained in a strainer lined with a paper coffee filter for 15 to 20 minutes, or ¼ cup fat-free sour cream

Lightly coat a large nonstick skillet with cooking spray. Add the onion, mushrooms, and bell pepper. Sauté over medium-high heat until they are softened and most of

(continued on page 148)

Grain Basics

Our supermarkets today are filled with healthful grains, full of nutrients and fiber. The ripened seed or fruit of cultivated grasses, grains are the world's most important staple food.

Here are the grains we've included in this book:

GRAIN	DESCRIPTION	LIQUID FOR EACH CUP OF DRY GRAIN	COOKING TIME (MINUTES)	YIELD
Barley				
pearl	bland flavor; soft texture	2 cups	45	2 cups
Buckwheat				
kasha	roasted, mild, nutty flavor	2 cups	12 to 15	2 cups
Corn				
cornmeal (polenta)	sweet taste; soft texture	4 cups	30 (4 to 5 for instant)	2 cups
grits	slightly sweet; soft texture	4 cups	15 to 20	4 cups
Millet				
	slightly nutty flavor; chewy texture	2½ cups	25 to 30	3½ cups
Quinoa				
	sweet flavor; soft texture	2 cups	15	3 cups
Rice				
white	bland flavor; soft texture	2 cups	20	3 cups
brown	nutty flavor; soft texture	1½ cups	30	3 cups
wild	intense nutty flavor; chewy texture	2½ cups	50 to 55	4 cups
Wheat				
bulgur	nutty flavor; soft texture	2 cups	20 to 25	2 cups
couscous (quick-cooking)	ground durum wheat	2 cups	3	3 cups

the liquid is evaporated, about 5 to 7 minutes. Transfer the mixture to a bowl and set aside.

Wipe out the skillet and again lightly coat with cooking spray. Toast the kasha over medium heat, stirring constantly, for 1 minute. Add the broth, bring to a simmer, and cover. Cook until all the broth has been absorbed, about 7 to 12 minutes—some brands cook more quickly than others.

Meanwhile, cook the pasta according to package directions. Drain and set aside. When the kasha is done, fluff with a fork and stir in the reserved cooked vegetables and pasta. Season with pepper.

Transfer to a serving bowl. Spoon yogurt around the edge and serve.

Makes 4 servings.

JOSLIN CHOICES: 2 carbohydrate (bread/starch)

PER SERVING: 181 calories (7% calories from fat), 2 g total fat (1 g saturated fat), 9 g protein, 36 g carbohydrates, 5 g dietary fiber, 2 mg cholesterol, 68 mg sodium, 267 mg potassium

Millet Cakes with Sun-Dried Tomatoes and Cheese over Greens

One doesn't usually think of millet when cooking grains; however, millet is a staple for almost one-third of the world's population, particularly in African and Asian countries. In several of our cookbooks, millet has come into play; here is one of the most savory dishes to date. Be sure your sun-dried tomatoes are dry-packed, not packed in oil.

These grain cakes are delicious by themselves or can be made smaller and served as a side dish in a larger meal.

> *2 tablespoons olive oil*
> *1 cup millet, rinsed and drained*
> *¼ cup minced red onion*
> *1 clove garlic, minced*
> *½ teaspoon crushed dried basil*
> *pinch saffron threads*

8 dry-packed sun-dried tomatoes, plumped in ¼ cup warm water for 5 minutes
2 cups canned low-fat, low-sodium chicken or vegetable broth
2 large eggs, lightly beaten, or ½ cup egg substitute
olive oil cooking spray
½ cup shredded reduced-fat mozzarella cheese
1 quart baby salad greens, including some arugula and radicchio, rinsed and dried

In a large heavy skillet, heat 1 tablespoon of the olive oil over medium heat. Add the millet and stir until the grains begin to color, 4 to 5 minutes. Scrape the millet into a bowl and return the skillet to the stove.

Add the remaining 1 tablespoon olive oil and the red onion and garlic. Cook, stirring, for 4 minutes, until the onion and garlic are limp. Stir in the basil and saffron. Drain the sun-dried tomatoes and finely dice. Add to the skillet along with the reserved millet and broth. Cover and cook, undisturbed, until the millet is done and all the liquid is absorbed, about 30 to 35 minutes.

Gently break up the grains with a fork and transfer to a large bowl. Stir in the beaten eggs. Using floured hands, form the millet mixture into 12 small cakes, about 2½ inches in diameter and ½ inch thick.

Lightly coat a large nonstick skillet with cooking spray. Add the millet cakes (you may need to do this in 2 batches) and cook, turning once, until crisp and golden brown on both sides, about 5 minutes per side. Top each cake with 2 teaspoons mozzarella, remove from the stove, cover the skillet, and let stand for a few minutes, until the cheese is melted.

Arrange the greens on 6 large plates. Top each with 2 hot millet cakes and serve at once.

Makes 6 servings.

JOSLIN CHOICES: 4 carbohydrate (bread/starch), 1 fat
PER SERVING: 415 calories (25% calories from fat), 11 g total fat (3 g saturated fat), 15 g
    protein, 63 g carbohydrates, 4 g dietary fiber, 77 mg cholesterol, 121 mg sodium, 329 mg
    potassium

Creamy Polenta with Vegetable Stew

*W*hen preparing polenta, make sure you use a deep nonstick pot: deep enough to prevent the bubbling hot cornmeal from burning you or sputtering all over your range.

In this recipe, we call for stone-ground cornmeal grits (the label also says polenta) for a more authentic flavor, like that of the polenta served in fine Italian restaurants. If you wish to shorten the cooking time, use instant polenta or finely ground cornmeal. It'll cook up in about 5 minutes, but the polenta flavor will be less intense.

VEGETABLE STEW
olive oil cooking spray
1 medium onion, chopped
2 large cloves garlic, minced
1 small eggplant, peeled and cut into cubes
1 small zucchini, sliced into ¼-inch-thick rounds
2 large tomatoes, cut into eighths
½ pound button mushrooms, halved if large
2 tablespoons chopped fresh basil
1 tablespoon chopped flat-leaf parsley
freshly ground pepper to taste

CREAMY POLENTA
3 to 4 cups water
1 cup stone-ground cornmeal grits (true polenta)
½ teaspoon salt (optional)
2 tablespoons grated Parmesan cheese

Lightly coat a nonstick pot with cooking spray and sauté the onion and garlic over medium heat for 2 minutes. Add the eggplant, zucchini, and tomatoes. Cover and simmer until the eggplant begins to soften, about 10 minutes. Add the mushrooms and continue to cook, uncovered, until all the vegetables are done, another 10 to 15 minutes. Stir in the basil, parsley, and pepper. Simmer for another 2 minutes.

Meanwhile, prepare the polenta. Bring 3 cups water to a boil. Reduce the heat to a simmer and stir in the cornmeal. Cook, stirring often, for 25 to 30 minutes, until thick and creamy, adding the remaining water if the polenta becomes too thick. It should resemble hot cereal. Add the salt and stir in the Parmesan cheese. Keep warm on the lowest heat or over a double boiler.

To serve, ladle the soft polenta into each of 4 shallow pasta bowls or large plates. Top with the vegetable stew and serve at once.

Makes 4 servings.

JOSLIN CHOICES: 3 carbohydrate (bread/starch)
PER SERVING: 253 calories (8% calories from fat), 2 g total fat (1 g saturated fat), 9 g protein, 52 g carbohydrates, 6 g dietary fiber, 2 mg cholesterol, 365 mg sodium, 884 mg potassium

Polenta Lasagna

*P*olenta has become a favorite of cooks everywhere. Here it's layered with fresh vegetables to make a rustic casserole that can be assembled ahead of time and baked when needed. If instant polenta isn't available in your store, substitute stone-ground yellow cornmeal.

butter-flavored cooking spray

SPINACH LAYER
2 shallots, minced
1 large clove garlic, minced
1 pound fresh spinach, well washed and tough stems discarded
2 tablespoons water
salt to taste (optional)
freshly ground pepper to taste

TOMATO LAYER
3 medium tomatoes, peeled, seeded, and chopped
1 tablespoon fresh thyme leaves or 1 teaspoon crushed dried

PORTOBELLO MUSHROOM LAYER

½ pound fresh portobello mushrooms, chopped

2 shallots, minced

1 tablespoon chopped fresh oregano or 1 teaspoon crushed dried

1 tablespoon dry white wine

POLENTA

4 cups canned low-fat, low-sodium chicken or vegetable broth

1 13-ounce package instant polenta

3 scallions, white part and 1 inch green, thinly sliced

2 tablespoons chopped flat-leaf parsley

⅓ cup freshly grated Parmesan cheese

Lightly coat a 10½ x 5 x 2½-inch loaf pan with cooking spray. Line the bottom and sides with parchment paper. Set aside.

To prepare the spinach layer, lightly coat a large nonstick skillet with cooking spray. Place over medium-low heat; add the shallots and garlic. Sauté, stirring often, until the shallots are limp but not browned.

Coarsely chop the spinach and add to the skillet along with the water, salt (if using), and pepper. Cook, stirring, until the spinach is wilted, about 2 minutes. Remove from the heat, transfer to a bowl, and set aside.

To prepare the tomato layer, coat the skillet with cooking spray. Add the tomatoes and thyme; cook, stirring frequently, until all liquid is evaporated, about 4 minutes. Transfer the mixture to a bowl and set aside.

To prepare the mushroom layer, coat the skillet with cooking spray. Add the mushrooms, shallots, and oregano. Cook, stirring, until the mushrooms are tender and the liquid is evaporated, about 5 minutes. Stir in the wine and cook, stirring, for 1 minute. Remove from the heat and set aside.

To prepare the polenta, in a large saucepan, bring the broth to a boil. Gradually whisk in the polenta, lower the heat, and cook, stirring, until the polenta is thickened, about 2 minutes. Whisk in the scallions, parsley, and Parmesan cheese. Remove from the heat.

To assemble, spoon one-quarter of the hot polenta mixture into the prepared loaf pan, smoothing the top with the back of a spoon. Top with the spinach mixture. Cover the spinach with another quarter of the polenta mixture. Top with the tomato mixture. Cover the tomatoes with the third quarter of polenta. Top with the mushroom mixture and then the remaining polenta mixture. Cover the pan with parchment paper. If making ahead, chill.

When ready to bake, preheat the oven to 350°F. Bake the lasagna until it is hot and set, about 30 to 45 minutes.

Remove from the oven and let stand for 5 minutes. Remove the top parchment paper and invert onto a serving platter. Remove the remaining parchment paper. Let stand about 10 minutes before slicing. Serve hot.

Makes 6 servings.

JOSLIN CHOICES: I very-low-fat protein, 3 carbohydrate (bread/starch)

PER SERVING: 305 calories (13% calories from fat), 5 g total fat (2 g saturated fat), 14 g
    protein, 54 g carbohydrates, 7 g dietary fiber, 7 mg cholesterol, 250 mg sodium, 756 mg
    potassium

Quinoa with Pineapple and Ginger

*W*e're lucky to live at a time when we have so many kinds of grains available at our supermarkets. Quinoa is an ancient mild-flavored, high-protein grain from the Andes of South America that was virtually unknown to the rest of the world not long ago. Today it's cultivated in Colorado and New Mexico and readily available at most supermarkets. You can also buy quinoa at health-food and organic markets.

> 1½ cups canned low-fat, low-sodium chicken or vegetable broth
> ½ teaspoon kosher salt (optional)
> 1 small bay leaf
> ¾ cup quinoa, rinsed and drained
> 1 teaspoon canola oil
> 3 tablespoons minced red onion
> 1 tablespoon finely grated fresh ginger
> 1 cup diced fresh pineapple (about ¼ pineapple)
> ¼ cup unsweetened or fresh pineapple juice
> 2 tablespoons fresh lime juice

2 tablespoons seasoned rice vinegar
1 tablespoon reduced-sodium soy sauce
1 teaspoon Thai or Vietnamese chili paste
1 teaspoon finely grated lime zest
1 bunch scallions, white part and 1 inch green, thinly sliced
⅓ cup finely chopped fresh mint or flat-leaf parsley

In a medium saucepan, bring the broth, salt (if using), and bay leaf to a rapid boil. Add the quinoa and stir. Reduce the heat to medium-low, cover, and simmer until the quinoa is tender, about 20 minutes. Remove from the heat and let stand for 10 minutes. Discard the bay leaf. Fluff the quinoa with a fork and set aside.

Meanwhile, heat the oil in a large nonstick skillet over low heat. Add the red onion, ginger, and pineapple. Sauté for 5 minutes, stirring frequently.

In a measuring cup, whisk together the pineapple juice, lime juice, rice vinegar, soy sauce, chili paste, and lime zest. Pour into the skillet and continue to cook, uncovered, until the mixture is thickened, about 6 to 7 minutes. Add the reserved quinoa and toss the mixture with 2 forks. Add the scallions and mint; toss again. Serve warm or cover and chill thoroughly before serving.

Makes 4 servings.

JOSLIN CHOICES: 2 carbohydrate (bread/starch)
PER SERVING: 187 calories (18% calories from fat), 4 g total fat (1 g saturated fat), 7 g
    protein, 34 g carbohydrates, 4 g dietary fiber, 1 mg cholesterol, 479 mg sodium, 436 mg
    potassium

Sushi

Sushi bars have spread across the country, even making their way into supermarkets. These Japanese delicacies are excellent for leftover bits and pieces of vegetables in your refrigerator. All you need is cooked short-grain rice, to which you add white wine or rice wine vinegar and a sugar substitute. This makes the sticky rice that holds the sushi together. You can then place some of the rice on a nori wrapper, top with thin slices of two or three vegetables, such as thin strips of carrot, paper-thin slices of seedless cucumber, thin strips of red or yellow bell pepper, tiny partially cooked tips of fresh asparagus, thin strips of scallion, and very thin slices of avocado. Add a bit of wasabi and roll it up. Mats to help you form tight rolls are available in most markets. You can also mold the rice, top with your favorite vegetables and tie with a bit of scallion. Make sure you have ice water nearby to dip your fingers and the rice mold in. This will keep the rice from sticking to your hands and the molds. The only thing left to do is to slice your sushi roll or decorate your small rice molds, place on lacquered plates with pickled ginger and more wasabi, and pass the chopsticks.

It is recommended that people with diabetes avoid eating raw fish or shellfish. If you are going to add bits of seafood to your sushi, make sure that you use only cooked pieces.

Sushi Glossary

Wasabi: a strong spice, unique to Japan, with a bright green color and flavor comparable to horseradish. Wasabi is hard to find fresh, but most markets carry powdered wasabi (reconstitute with water) or wasabi paste. Use as a "glue" to stick the vegetables to the rice, or mix with a little reduced-sodium soy sauce for dipping the finished sushi.

Nori: seaweed that has been stretched on bamboo frames to dry in sheets. Sold ten to a package in Asian markets and many supermarkets, nori is used when making rolled sushi. The shiny side should be on the outside, the rough side next to the filling.

Pickled ginger: a palate cleanser, these pink strips of breathtaking gingerroot should be eaten between pieces of sushi.

Sticky Rice for Sushi

2 cups sushi (short-grain jasmine) rice
2 cups water
1 teaspoon salt (optional)
⅓ cup rice wine vinegar

Wash the rice in a colander until the water is clear, about 3 to 5 minutes. Place in a heavy saucepan with 2 cups water. Cover and bring to a boil over high heat. Reduce the heat to medium and boil for 5 minutes. Reduce the heat to low and continue cooking for another 15 minutes. DO NOT remove the lid while cooking. Remove from the heat and set aside.

Combine the salt (if using) and vinegar. Slowly stir the vinegar mixture into the rice, coating all of the grains. Allow the rice to stand until cool enough to touch.

Makes enough for 10 rolls.

JOSLIN CHOICES (per roll): 2 carbohydrate (bread/starch)
PER SERVING: 136 calories (0% from fat), 0 total fat (0 saturated fat), 2 g protein, 30 g
carbohydrates, 1 g dietary fiber, 0 cholesterol, 123 mg sodium, 0 potassium

Basmati Rice with Black Beans and Mango

This is so good that you'll want to prepare it often, substituting other fresh fruit of the season for the mango—oranges in the winter, strawberries in the spring, or papaya or peaches in the summer.

1 cup basmati rice
1 15-ounce can black beans, rinsed well and drained
⅛ teaspoon crushed red pepper flakes
¼ teaspoon salt (optional)
3 tablespoons fresh orange juice
2 teaspoons grated orange zest

¼ cup chopped fresh cilantro
2 teaspoons minced fresh ginger
½ teaspoon ground cumin
vegetable cooking spray
3 scallions, white part and 1 inch green, chopped
2 cloves garlic, minced
1 small red bell pepper, seeded and cut into thin julienne strips
1 large ripe mango, peeled and cut into thin slices (see page 56)

Prepare the rice according to package directions. When done, stir in the black beans, red pepper flakes, salt (if using), orange juice, zest, cilantro, ginger, and cumin. Keep warm.

Lightly coat a nonstick skillet with cooking spray. Sauté the scallions, garlic, and bell pepper until soft, about 4 minutes. Add to the rice and fold in the mango. Serve immediately.

Makes 6 servings.

JOSLIN CHOICES: 3 carbohydrate (2 bread/starch, 1 fruit)
PER SERVING: 211 calories (5% calories from fat), 1 g total fat (0 saturated fat), 7 g protein,
44 g carbohydrates, 5 g dietary fiber, 0 cholesterol, 318 mg sodium, 125 mg potassium

Confetti Risotto

*T*his Italian rice dish is made with short-grain rice that, when cooked properly, has a tender, creamy texture. Make sure to keep the broth simmering and serve the risotto piping hot.

1 tablespoon olive oil
1 medium onion, chopped
2 large cloves garlic, minced
1 cup Arborio or Carnaroli (Italian short-grain) rice
½ cup dry white wine
3 cups canned low-fat, low-sodium chicken or vegetable broth

½ cup water

3 medium plum tomatoes, seeded and chopped

1 medium yellow tomato, seeded and chopped

3 tablespoons minced fresh basil

2 tablespoons grated Parmesan cheese

Heat the oil in a nonstick pot and sauté the onion and garlic for 2 minutes over low heat. Add the rice and stir for another 2 minutes. Stir in the wine, raise the heat to medium, and cook, stirring, until the liquid has been absorbed.

Meanwhile, in a large pot, bring the broth and water to a slow simmer. Ladle 1 cup stock into the rice and cook at a simmer, stirring, until most of the broth has been absorbed. Add the remaining broth, ½ cup at a time, continuing to stir until the rice is al dente, about 25 minutes total cooking time. Stir in the tomatoes, basil, and Parmesan cheese. Serve immediately.

Makes 4 servings.

JOSLIN CHOICES: 3 carbohydrate (bread/starch), I vegetable, I fat

PER SERVING: 328 calories (16% calories from fat), 6 g total fat (2 g saturated fat), 9 g
protein, 53 g carbohydrates, 2 g dietary fiber, 5 mg cholesterol, 336 mg sodium, 328 mg
potassium

Risotto Tips

Don't rinse the rice or other grain before cooking; the surface starch on every grain is necessary for making a creamy risotto.

Be sure to use a heavy pot that heats evenly. The sides of the pot should be straight and the bottom flat to allow for even cooking.

Keep both broth and the risotto cooking at a lively simmer so that the risotto cooks properly. If adding vegetables, sauté briefly and add at the end so that they don't become overcooked.

Usually the total cooking time for risotto will be about 25 to 30 minutes, but start testing for doneness after about 15 minutes of total cooking time. Remember, the risotto is done when its texture is the way you like it.

Fried Rice with Tofu

*M*aking fried rice is one of the tastiest ways of using leftovers we know. Bring out all those dabs of cooked veggies from the refrigerator, add a bit of tofu plus some cooked rice, and in a matter of minutes, you'll have a meal.

1 tablespoon vegetable oil

1 medium onion, chopped

3 cloves garlic, minced

1½-inch piece fresh ginger, peeled and minced

4 ounces mushrooms, sliced

3 cups leftover or fresh cooked vegetables (such as broccoli, asparagus, peas, or green beans), cut into bite-size pieces

4 ounces firm tofu, drained and pressed, cut into bite-size pieces (page 179)

2 cups cooked rice

1 tablespoon reduced-sodium soy sauce

¼ cup canned low-fat, low-sodium chicken or vegetable broth

1 tablespoon dry sherry

¼ cup egg substitute

2 scallions, white part and 1 inch green, thinly sliced, for garnish (optional)

Heat the oil in a nonstick wok or heavy skillet until it is hot but not smoking. Add the onion, garlic, ginger, and mushrooms. Stir-fry for 3 to 4 minutes, until the onion begins to wilt. Add the vegetables and tofu; stir-fry for 2 minutes.

Add the rice, soy sauce, broth, and sherry. Stir-fry for 2 more minutes. Push the rice-vegetable mixture to one side of the wok. Add the egg substitute to the free space in the wok and stir-fry it quickly. As it cooks, gradually stir the rice mixture into the eggs. Garnish with scallions (if desired). Serve at once.

Makes 4 servings.

JOSLIN CHOICES: 2 carbohydrate (bread/starch), I fat

PER SERVING: 198 calories (25% calories from fat), 6 g total fat (I g saturated fat), 9 g protein, 29 g carbohydrates, 4 g dietary fiber, 0 cholesterol, 184 mg sodium, 513 mg potassium

Spices, Herbs, and Other Seasonings for Rice

parsley, dill, tarragon, chervil, mint

scallions

Parmesan cheese

toasted nuts

currants, raisins, dried cherries, and
    dried apricots

garlic

grated zest of lemon, lime, or orange

ginger, grated fresh or ground

bell and chile peppers

sun-dried tomatoes

basil, onion, and chopped tomatoes

saffron

mushrooms

sunflower seeds

sesame seeds

reduced-sodium soy sauce

Spanish Vegetable and Rice Medley

We first tasted this delicious rice medley at the midnight buffet of the Costa Lines cruise ship *Carla C* after an evening performance of flamenco dancers on shore in Palma de Majorca. We begged the chef for the recipe, which is perfect for a light snack. Since we're cooking with less fat, we reduced the olive oil in his recipe and discarded the egg yolks from the hard-cooked eggs. The result is an even lighter mixture that still is as delicious as we remember.

DRESSING

2 shallots, minced

1 clove garlic, minced

1 tablespoon minced flat-leaf parsley

1 tablespoon Dijon mustard

3 tablespoons red wine vinegar

3 tablespoons olive oil

1 tablespoon fat-free sour cream

2 hard-cooked egg whites, chopped

VEGETABLES AND RICE
3 medium tomatoes, cut into 6 wedges
2 medium green bell peppers, seeded and cut into thin julienne strips
½ small red onion, thinly sliced
½ pound tiny green beans, blanched in boiling water 1 minute and drained
1 cup cooked brown rice

In a small bowl, combine the shallots, garlic, and parsley. Add the mustard, vinegar, and oil. Whisk thoroughly. While still whisking, incorporate the sour cream and egg whites to form a dressing. Set aside.

In a large bowl, combine the vegetables and rice, mixing gently. Pour the dressing over the mixture. Mix well and serve.

Makes 6 servings.

JOSLIN CHOICES: 1 carbohydrate (bread/starch), 2 fat
PER SERVING: 156 calories (42% calories from fat), 8 g total fat (1 g saturated fat), 4 g protein,
    20 g carbohydrates, 4 g dietary fiber, 0 cholesterol, 113 mg sodium, 390 mg potassium

A Touch of Green

*Y*ou'll notice that we never give a dried equivalent for parsley—simply because dried parsley has neither the bright color nor the marvelous flavor of fresh parsley and is, in our opinion, a waste of money. Fortunately, both the common curly parsley and the more intensely flavored flat-leaf parsley freeze well. The former is used as a garnish and the latter in recipes, since flat-leaf parsley holds up well in cooking.

Dirt and grit can hide in the leaves of parsley, so it's essential to wash it before chopping and freezing. An easy way to wash parsley (and other green herbs) is to immerse it in bunches in cold water, holding the stems and swishing the leaves vigorously. Repeat in a clean batch of water until the water remains clear. Air-dry on paper towels for at least 30 minutes, then chop (a food processor makes quick work of this task). If the chopped parsley seems damp, again air-dry on paper towels. Then transfer the chopped parsley to plastic freezer containers and freeze. The parsley can be measured into spoons or cups without thawing.

Southwestern Tabbouleh

*W*e've taken liberties with tabbouleh, which is essentially a Middle Eastern parsley salad, by adding vegetables and flavors of our own Southwest. The result is a lively combination, equally welcome for hot or cold weather meals.

1 cup water

½ cup low-sodium vegetable juice

1 teaspoon ground cumin

½ teaspoon salt (optional)

⅛ teaspoon freshly ground black pepper

⅛ teaspoon cayenne pepper

1 cup bulgur wheat

1 cup frozen corn kernels, thawed and drained

2 large plum tomatoes, seeded and diced

1 small red onion, finely diced

1 small green bell pepper, seeded and finely diced

1 small cucumber, seeded and finely diced

1 small fresh jalapeño chile pepper, seeded and finely diced

2 cups chopped flat-leaf parsley

¼ cup chopped fresh cilantro

DRESSING

½ cup fresh lemon juice

3 tablespoons olive oil

2 large cloves garlic, finely minced

⅛ teaspoon hot pepper sauce

small inner romaine lettuce leaves

In a large pot, combine the water, vegetable juice, cumin, salt (if using), black pepper, and cayenne pepper. Bring to a boil over medium-high heat. Cook, stirring, for 1 minute. Remove from the heat and stir in the bulgur. Cover and let stand until the bulgur absorbs the liquid, about 1 hour.

Fluff the bulgur with a fork and transfer to a large salad bowl. Add the corn, tomatoes, onion, bell pepper, cucumber, and chile pepper. Sprinkle with the parsley and cilantro. Toss gently to combine well.

To make the dressing, in a small bowl whisk together the lemon juice, oil, garlic, and hot pepper sauce. Drizzle over the bulgur mixture and toss again. Cover and refrigerate for at least 4 hours before serving. Mound the tabbouleh in a shallow serving dish and surround with lettuce leaves. Serve cold or at room temperature.

Makes 6 servings.

JOSLIN CHOICES: 1 carbohydrate (bread/starch), 2 vegetable, 1 fat
PER SERVING: 203 calories (32% calories from fat), 8 g total fat (1 g saturated fat), 6 g
    protein, 32 g carbohydrates, 7 g dietary fiber, 0 cholesterol, 231 mg sodium, 479 mg
    potassium

Sweet-and-Sour Stuffed Cabbage Rolls

*T*he memories that accompany this recipe run deep into childhood, with dinners around the family table and at ethnic restaurants in New York. Try making the stuffed rolls with brown rice seasoned with a bit of fresh dill. You can't go wrong.

vegetable cooking spray
1 medium onion, chopped
1 large portobello mushroom, diced
¾ cup long-grain white rice
1¾ cups boiling water
¼ teaspoon salt (optional)
freshly ground pepper to taste
¼ cup egg substitute
10 large cabbage leaves
1 28-ounce can no-salt-added crushed tomatoes
1 medium carrot, grated
2 tablespoons dried currants

1 packet sugar substitute
3 tablespoons fresh lemon juice

Lightly coat a covered nonstick pot with cooking spray. Sauté half of the chopped onion with the mushroom pieces until the onion begins to soften, about 4 minutes. Add the rice and stir to coat. Add the water, cover, and simmer until the rice is done and the liquid is absorbed, about 20 to 25 minutes. Add the salt (if using), pepper, and egg substitute. Stir over low heat for 1 minute. Set aside.

Bring a large kettle of water to a boil. Core the cabbage and place in the pot. Simmer for 5 minutes. Remove and, starting at the core end, carefully pull off 10 leaves. With a sharp knife, cut out the thick center of each leaf. Chop 2 of the remaining cabbage leaves and set aside.

Pour the crushed tomatoes into a large nonstick pot with a cover. Stir in the carrot, reserved chopped cabbage, remaining onions, currants, sugar substitute, and lemon juice. Simmer over low heat while you stuff the cabbage leaves.

Place the cabbage leaves on a large work surface. Put 3 tablespoons of the rice mixture at the bottom of each leaf and roll up, folding in the sides and completely enclosing the filling. Place the cabbage rolls, seam down, in the simmering tomato sauce. Spoon some of the sauce over the cabbage rolls. Cover and simmer slowly for 1 hour, adding more water if necessary. Serve hot.

Makes 4 servings.

JOSLIN CHOICES: 2 carbohydrate (bread/starch), 2 vegetable
PER SERVING: 250 calories (6% calories from fat), 2 g total fat (0 saturated fat), 10 g protein,
  50 g carbohydrates, 8 g dietary fiber, 0 cholesterol, 683 mg sodium, 397 mg potassium

Vegetable Paella

Sometimes we can buy baby artichokes about the size of an egg in our supermarket. Sold by the weight, these artichokes have not developed the inedible fuzzy choke in the center, so once the outside leaves are trimmed away, the entire artichoke is edible.

If you can't find baby artichokes, buy two globe or large ones. Slice off the top third of each artichoke and remove the outer leaves until you reach the tender center leaves.

Quarter the artichokes and, using a spoon, scoop out and discard the fuzzy choke. Leave the tender inner core of the artichoke intact.

8 baby artichokes
lemon water made with juice of 1 lemon and 2 cups water
3 fresh sage leaves
1 teaspoon grated lemon zest
1 clove garlic, peeled
olive oil cooking spray
1 small red onion, chopped
1 medium red bell pepper, seeded and chopped
2 cloves garlic, minced
1½ cups long-grain white rice
1 15-ounce can chickpeas, rinsed well and drained
1½ cups canned low-fat, low-sodium chicken or vegetable broth
1½ cups water
¾ teaspoon saffron threads
¼ teaspoon salt (optional)
freshly ground pepper to taste
1 cup frozen baby peas
2 tablespoons thinly sliced black olives for garnish (optional)
3 tablespoons chopped fresh cilantro or mint for garnish (optional)

Remove the tough outer layer of leaves from the artichokes. Cut off the stems and, if using them, peel and slice. Immediately immerse in lemon water to keep the artichokes' bright color while you're trimming the rest.

Place the artichokes and lemon water in a covered pot. Add the sage, lemon zest, and peeled garlic. Bring to a boil, lower the heat, cover, and simmer until the artichokes are tender, about 15 minutes. Drain and set aside.

Lightly coat a large nonstick skillet or paella pan with cooking spray. Sauté the onion, bell pepper, and minced garlic for 3 minutes. Add the rice and chickpeas, along with the broth, water, saffron, salt (if using), and pepper. Bring to a boil and simmer, uncovered, until the rice is cooked, about 18 minutes, adding the peas during the last 5 minutes of cooking time. Place the artichokes on top of the rice and garnish with the olives and cilantro or mint (if using).

Makes 6 servings.

JOSLIN CHOICES: 4 carbohydrate (bread/starch)

PER SERVING: 389 calories (8% calories from fat), 4 g total fat (1 g saturated fat), 15 g
protein, 79 g carbohydrates, 16 g dietary fiber, 1 mg cholesterol, 588 mg sodium, 955 mg
potassium

Wild and White Rice with Winter Fruits

*N*ative Americans have been gathering true native wild rice the same way for hundreds of years in the glacier-carved wetlands north of Minneapolis, Minnesota. Traveling in pairs in their wooden canoes, one person poles from the stern while the other uses cedar sticks to pull the tall stalks of aquatic grass over the sides of the boat and knock the ripe grains loose. Back on shore, the grains are first dried in the sun, then put into an iron kettle over a roaring wood fire. The hulling and winnowing, once done by hand, are now done by machine. Connoisseurs can tell the difference between true native wild rice and the commonly sold cultivated wild rice. If it's not harvested manually, it must, by law, say "cultivated wild rice" on the label. Either kind will work in this recipe. This recipe combines wild and white rices with winter fruits for exceptional taste and texture.

4 cups cold water
1 cup wild rice, rinsed and drained
1 tablespoon olive oil
1 cup diced red onion
1 cup diced celery
2 cups long-grain white rice
4½ cups canned low-fat, low-sodium chicken or vegetable broth
2 medium navel oranges
1 cup no-sugar-added dried cherries
1 teaspoon crushed dried thyme
¼ cup chopped fresh mint or flat-leaf parsley

In a heavy saucepan, bring the water to a boil over high heat. Stir in the wild rice, reduce the heat, and simmer, uncovered, until just tender, 30 to 45 minutes. Do not overcook. Drain, set aside, and keep warm.

In the same saucepan, heat the olive oil over medium-low heat. Add the red onion and celery. Sauté, stirring occasionally, until the vegetables are limp but not brown, about 4 minutes. Stir in the white rice and add the broth. Bring the mixture to a boil.

Reduce the heat, cover, and simmer for 20 minutes, until the rice is tender. Fluff with a fork and stir in the reserved wild rice. Set aside and keep warm.

Grate the zest from the oranges and add to the rice mixture. Working over a bowl to catch any juice, peel the oranges, removing all the white pith. Section the oranges and add to the rice mixture. Stir the dried cherries into any accumulated orange juice, then add the cherries to the rice mixture. Stir in the thyme and mint. Serve warm.

Makes 12 servings.

JOSLIN CHOICES: 3 carbohydrate (2 bread/starch, 1 fruit)
PER SERVING: 240 calories (8% calories from fat), 2 g total fat (1 g saturated fat), 6 g protein,
48 g carbohydrates, 3 g dietary fiber, 1 mg cholesterol, 55 mg sodium, 191 mg potassium

Beans, Legumes, and Tofu

Cannellini Balsamico

In Tuscany this classic bean dish is often cooked overnight in an empty Chianti bottle buried in the embers of a hearth. We cook ours on top of the stove and use the best balsamic vinegar that we can afford. These are lovely as a side dish or great as a light meal with a crisp green salad.

½ pound dried cannellini beans, rinsed and picked over, then soaked or quick-soaked (see box, page 168)

1 small white onion, minced
1 large clove garlic, minced
2 tablespoons fresh thyme leaves or 2 teaspoons crushed dried
3 tablespoons chopped flat-leaf parsley
2 tablespoons olive oil
1 tablespoon balsamic vinegar
1 teaspoon salt (optional)
freshly ground pepper to taste

Fill a pot with cold water to cover the beans by 2 inches. Bring to a boil. Reduce the heat and partially cover. Cook the beans for 1 to 1½ hours, or until tender, keeping the beans covered with water during the cooking period.

When the beans are done, drain and place them in a large bowl. Stir in the remaining ingredients, including the salt (if using) and pepper. Let stand for at least 30 minutes before serving warm or at room temperature.

Makes 4 servings.

JOSLIN CHOICES: 1 low-fat protein, 1½ carbohydrate (bread/starch)
PER SERVING: 243 calories (15% calories from fat), 4 g total fat (1 g saturated fat), 13 g
   protein, 40 g carbohydrates, 16 g dietary fiber, 0 cholesterol, 11 mg sodium, 945 mg
   potassium

Quick-Soaking Beans

If you forgot to soak dried beans the night before, you can always use the quick-soak method.

Put the beans in a large pot, covered by 2 inches of cold water. Bring to a boil over medium-high heat. Boil for 2 minutes. Remove from the heat and let stand for 1 hour, covered. Drain the beans and rinse in several changes of cold water. Drain again. The beans are now ready to cook.

Refried Spicy Black Beans

Next time you're serving Tex-Mex food, try these spicy refried beans. We first sampled this bean "pancake" in a Cuban restaurant in Miami Beach, and now we frequently make individual portions to serve with the occasional poached egg on top for Sunday brunch.

olive oil cooking spray
1 tablespoon olive oil
1 small red bell pepper, seeded and minced
1 small onion, minced
3 large cloves garlic, minced
1 small jalapeño chile pepper, seeded and minced
3 cups cooked black beans
3 scallions, white part only, minced
½ teaspoon ground cumin
½ teaspoon crushed dried oregano, preferably Mexican
salt to taste (optional)
freshly ground pepper to taste
¼ cup fat-free sour cream
¼ cup minced fresh cilantro

Lightly coat a 10-inch nonstick skillet with cooking spray. Add the olive oil and place over medium-low heat. Add the bell pepper, onion, garlic, and chile pepper. Sauté, stirring often, until the vegetables are limp, about 5 minutes.

Stir in the black beans, scallions, cumin, and oregano. Season with salt (if using) and pepper. Cook over medium heat for 5 minutes, gently mashing the beans with a pancake turner to form a compact cake.

Reduce the heat to low and continue to cook another 10 to 15 minutes, until the bottom is crusty and a thick pancake has formed. Invert onto a serving platter and top with dollops of sour cream. Sprinkle with cilantro and serve at once.

Makes 4 servings.

JOSLIN CHOICES: 1 low-fat protein, 1½ carbohydrate (bread/starch)

PER SERVING: 173 calories (16% calories from fat), 4 g total fat (0 saturated fat), 12 g protein, 32 g carbohydrates, 10 g dietary fiber, 1 mg cholesterol, 406 mg sodium, 663 mg potassium

Black-eyed Pea Jambalaya

*J*ambalaya is a one-dish Creole meal that's beloved by those who live in Louisiana and surrounding states, as well as by untold others elsewhere. It's usually made with whatever ingredients are on hand, but every version includes rice. Our vegetable version revolves around a base of black-eyed peas with specks of brightly colored vegetables and rice. Jambalaya tastes great the day it's made—and even better the next day. Don't forget to pass several bottles of different hot sauces for adding at the last minute.

1 tablespoon canola oil

1 large onion, chopped

2 large cloves garlic, minced

½ cup finely diced celery

½ cup finely diced carrots

1 large green bell pepper, seeded and finely diced

1 large red bell pepper, seeded and finely diced

1 teaspoon crushed dried thyme

2 teaspoons paprika

salt to taste (optional)

½ teaspoon lemon pepper

⅛ teaspoon cayenne pepper

2 cups cooked black-eyed peas

1 28-ounce can no-salt-added diced tomatoes with juice

3½ cups canned low-fat, low-sodium chicken or vegetable broth

½ tablespoon Worcestershire sauce

1 cup long-grain white rice

¼ cup chopped flat-leaf parsley

bottles of hot pepper sauce

In a heavy nonstick pot, heat the oil over medium heat. Add the onion, garlic, celery, and carrots. Cook, stirring, until the vegetables are limp, about 5 minutes. Add the bell peppers, thyme, paprika, salt (if using), lemon pepper, and cayenne pepper. Cook, continuing to stir occasionally, until the bell peppers are tender, about 5 minutes.

Stir in the black-eyed peas, tomatoes and their juice, broth, and Worcestershire sauce. Cook, partially covered, for 10 minutes, until the flavors blend. Add the rice and cook, covered, until the rice is tender, about 15 minutes.

Stir in the parsley and serve. Pass several kinds of hot pepper sauce to sprinkle on each serving.

Makes 8 servings.

JOSLIN CHOICES: 2 carbohydrate (bread/starch)

PER SERVING: 211 calories (13% calories from fat), 3 g total fat (1 g saturated fat), 8 g protein, 38 g carbohydrates, 6 g dietary fiber, 2 mg cholesterol, 123 mg sodium, 419 mg potassium

Cuban Black Beans over Broiled Papaya

Several Cuban restaurants in Miami serve this dish. We love the spiciness of the beans contrasted with the sweetness of the papaya. It's terrific served by itself as a light lunch or alongside other foods as a side dish.

½ pound dried black beans, rinsed and picked over, then soaked or quick-soaked (page 168)

3 cups cold water

1 tablespoon olive oil

1 large yellow onion, chopped

1 medium green bell pepper, seeded and chopped

2 large cloves garlic, minced

½ teaspoon ground cumin

½ teaspoon crushed dried oregano

1 small bay leaf
2 teaspoons light brown sugar
1 teaspoon salt (optional)
¼ teaspoon freshly ground pepper
½ tablespoon red wine vinegar
1 large papaya
¼ cup minced fresh cilantro

Put the beans in a large pot with the water. Bring to a boil over high heat. Reduce the heat to low and simmer, uncovered, until the beans are barely tender, about 30 minutes. Skim off and discard any foam that rises to the surface.

Meanwhile, heat the oil in a large nonstick skillet over medium-low heat. Add the onion, bell pepper, and garlic. Sauté, stirring occasionally, until the onion is limp, about 5 minutes. Stir in the cumin, oregano, bay leaf, and ½ teaspoon of the brown sugar.

Set a colander over a large bowl and drain the beans, reserving 1½ cups of the cooking liquid. Return the beans and reserved cooking liquid to the pot, along with the sautéed onion mixture. Cook, uncovered, for another 30 minutes, stirring occasionally. Add the salt (if using) and pepper. Remove the bay leaf and stir in the vinegar.

Slice off the stem end of the papaya. Using a spoon, carefully remove and discard the seeds. Peel the papaya and cut crosswise into 4 thick slices.

When the beans are done, preheat the broiler and position the rack 6 inches from the source of the heat.

Place the papaya slices on a baking sheet and sprinkle with the remaining 1½ teaspoons brown sugar. Broil until the papaya is heated through and the sugar begins to bubble and brown. Using a spatula, transfer the papaya slices to a serving platter. Top with hot black beans and sprinkle with cilantro. Serve at once.

Makes 4 servings.

JOSLIN CHOICES: 1 very-low-fat protein, 2 carbohydrate (bread/starch), 1 vegetable
PER SERVING: 281 calories (13% calories from fat), 4 g total fat (1 g saturated fat), 14 g
    protein, 50 g carbohydrates, 14 g dietary fiber, 0 cholesterol, 20 mg sodium, 923 mg
    potassium

Chickpeas and Tomatoes, Persian-Style

*O*ur Persian friend Parvine has always teased us about our restrained use of dried herbs by the quarter, half, or full teaspoon. When cooking her native foods, she thinks that the more herbs, the better the dish. We agreed when we tasted this chickpea dish—the dried herbs may seem like an excessive amount, but they mellow out in cooking to produce a very pleasing dish.

½ pound dried chickpeas, rinsed and picked over
3 tablespoons chopped flat-leaf parsley
2 tablespoons crushed dried cilantro
2 tablespoons crushed dried mint
1 tablespoon crushed dried tarragon
olive oil cooking spray
1 medium onion, halved and thinly sliced
1 28-ounce can no-salt-added plum tomatoes with juice, chopped
2 tablespoons golden raisins
1 teaspoon grated lemon zest
½ teaspoon turmeric
1 pound fresh spinach, washed well and drained, tough stems discarded
salt to taste (optional)
freshly ground pepper to taste

In a large bowl, soak the chickpeas overnight in cold water to cover. Drain and place in a large saucepan along with the parsley, cilantro, mint, tarragon, and fresh water to cover by 2 inches. Partially cover and simmer, adding more water if necessary, for 1 to 1¼ hours, until the chickpeas are barely tender. Remove from the heat (recipe may be made ahead to this point, covered, and refrigerated overnight). Do not drain.

Lightly coat a large nonstick skillet with cooking spray. Add the onion and cook, stirring occasionally, until limp, about 4 minutes. Add the tomatoes with their juice, chickpeas with their cooking liquid, and the raisins, lemon zest, and turmeric. Bring to a slow simmer. Partially cover and simmer for 45 minutes, until the chickpeas are tender and the liquid is slightly thickened. Stir in the spinach and cook until it wilts, another 1 to 2 minutes. Taste and season with salt (if using) and pepper. Transfer to a large serving bowl. Serve at once.

Makes 4 servings.

JOSLIN CHOICES: 1 very-low-fat protein, 2½ carbohydrate (bread/starch)

PER SERVING: 308 calories (12% calories from fat), 4 g total fat (0 saturated fat), 18 g protein, 55 g carbohydrates, 17 g dietary fiber, 0 cholesterol, 134 mg sodium, 1,684 mg potassium

Lentils with Spinach

You can also make this Middle Eastern dish with Swiss chard, broccoli rabe, or even mustard greens in place of the spinach.

½ pound dried brown lentils, rinsed and picked over
1 large leek, trimmed, cleaned, and sliced
1 small onion, chopped
3 large cloves garlic, minced
3 cups water
1 small bay leaf
salt to taste (optional)
freshly ground pepper to taste
1 pound fresh spinach, well washed and tough stems discarded
1 teaspoon ground cumin
½ teaspoon ground coriander
juice of ½ lemon

In a saucepan, combine the lentils, leek, onion, garlic, water, and bay leaf. Bring to a boil. Reduce the heat, cover, and simmer for 30 minutes, until the lentils are tender. Season with salt (if using) and pepper.

Chop the spinach and place in a large nonstick skillet. Wilt over medium heat in its own liquid. Drain the lentils, reserving some of the cooking liquid. Discard the bay leaf. Add the lentil mixture to the spinach, along with the cumin and coriander.

Stir together over medium heat for 5 minutes, adding more lentil cooking liquid if the mixture becomes too dry. Squeeze lemon juice over all and serve hot.

Makes 4 servings.

JOSLIN CHOICES: 2 very-low-fat protein, 1½ carbohydrate (bread/starch)
PER SERVING: 249 calories (4% calories from fat), 1 g total fat (0 saturated fat), 20 g protein,
    44 g carbohydrates, 22 g dietary fiber, 0 cholesterol, 102 mg sodium, 1,261 mg potassium

Texas Pot of Pintos

*W*here we live, beans are a popular potluck supper dish, especially pinto beans. Here they are served Texas-style, with lots of onion, garlic, and hot seasonings. Don't add any salt (if using) until the end, as it prevents the beans from becoming tender as they cook.

1 cup dried pinto beans, rinsed and picked over, then soaked or quick-soaked (page 168)
6 cups water
1 large bay leaf
2 cups chopped onion
4 large cloves garlic, peeled
1 large fresh jalapeño chile pepper (optional)
2 cups canned low-fat, low-sodium chicken or vegetable broth
½ tablespoon good-quality chili powder
1 teaspoon freshly ground black pepper
¼ teaspoon cayenne pepper
½ teaspoon salt, or to taste (optional)
¼ cup chopped fresh cilantro

Place the beans in a large pot; add the water and bay leaf. Bring to a boil and boil for 10 minutes, skimming off any foam that rises to the surface. Lower the heat and add the onion, garlic, jalapeño (if using), broth, chili powder, black pepper, and cayenne pepper. Cover and cook until the beans are tender, 1½ to 2 hours.

When the beans are tender, add the salt (if using) and remove the bay leaf and discard. If a thicker broth is desired, use the back of a large spoon to crush some of the cooked pintos against the side of the pot. Stir the mashed pintos back into the mixture. Repeat until the desired thickness is obtained.

Just before serving, sprinkle with cilantro. Serve hot.

Makes 4 servings.

JOSLIN CHOICES: 1 very-low-fat protein, 2 carbohydrate (bread/starch)

PER SERVING: 220 calories (7% calories from fat), 2 g total fat (1 g saturated fat), 13 g
protein, 41 g carbohydrates, 12 g dietary fiber, 2 mg cholesterol, 360 mg sodium, 723 mg
potassium

White Beans, Peasant-Style

*T*his recipe skips the usual soaking time yet results in a perfectly tender bean. Use this cooking technique to shorten other recipes with dried beans.

1 cup dried white beans, rinsed and picked over
6 cups cold water
1 large bay leaf
1 tablespoon olive oil
½ small red onion, thinly sliced
2 large cloves garlic, thinly sliced
1 tablespoon fresh thyme leaves or 1 teaspoon crushed dried
1 tablespoon chopped fresh basil or 1 teaspoon crushed dried
2 cups canned low-fat, low-sodium chicken or vegetable broth
12 large cherry tomatoes, quartered
½ teaspoon salt (optional)
freshly ground pepper to taste
2 tablespoons chopped flat-leaf parsley

Place the beans in a large pot and add the water and bay leaf. Bring to a boil and boil for 10 minutes, skimming off any foam that rises to the surface. Lower the heat, cover, and cook until the beans are tender, 45 minutes to 1 hour. Drain and discard the bay leaf. Set the beans aside.

Rinse and dry the pot. Add the olive oil and place over medium heat. Add the red onion and garlic. Cook, stirring frequently, until the onion and garlic are limp but not browned, about 4 to 5 minutes. Stir in the thyme, basil, and broth. Return the reserved beans to the pot and add the tomatoes. Stir to mix. Cook for another 3 to 4 minutes, until the tomatoes begin to wilt. Transfer the beans to a serving bowl and season with salt (if using) and pepper. Sprinkle with parsley. Serve at once.

Makes 4 servings.

JOSLIN CHOICES: 1 medium-fat protein, 1½ carbohydrate (bread/starch)
PER SERVING: 239 calories (19% calories from fat), 5 g total fat (1 g saturated fat), 13 g
protein, 37 g carbohydrates, 14 g dietary fiber, 2 mg cholesterol, 355 mg sodium, 720 mg
potassium

Spicy Tofu and Chinese Vegetables

*T*he black bean sauce, chili puree with garlic, five-spice powder, and Chinese cooking wine needed for this savory dish are all available in supermarkets or specialty stores. The recipe is high in sodium, so make sure it fits within your meal plan, especially if you're on a sodium-restricted diet.

12 ounces firm tofu, pressed and weighted, then cut into 1 x ¼-inch slices (see page 179)
3 tablespoons Chinese cooking wine
1 tablespoon reduced-sodium soy sauce
⅛ teaspoon dark sesame oil
½ teaspoon five-spice powder
½ cup canned low-fat, low-sodium chicken or vegetable broth
1 tablespoon cornstarch
1 tablespoon canola oil
1 tablespoon black bean sauce
2 teaspoons chili puree with garlic

⅛ *teaspoon sugar substitute*
1 medium red bell pepper, seeded and cut into thin julienne strips
¼ *pound snow peas, strings removed*
½ *pound bean sprouts*
2 scallions, white part only, thinly sliced

Place the tofu in a flat dish. Combine 1½ tablespoons of the cooking wine, 1 teaspoon of the soy sauce, and the sesame oil and five-spice powder. Pour over the tofu. Marinate at least 1 hour or overnight.

Preheat the broiler. Transfer the tofu to a paper towel to drain. Broil until lightly browned and crisp. Set aside.

In a small cup, combine the broth and cornstarch. Set aside.

Heat the oil in a large nonstick skillet over medium heat. Add the black bean sauce, chili puree with garlic, and sugar substitute. Stir for a minute to combine. Add the bell pepper, snow peas, remaining 1½ tablespoons cooking wine, and remaining 2 teaspoons soy sauce. Cook over high heat until the snow peas are just about done, about 2 minutes. Add the bean sprouts and scallions along with the broth and cornstarch mixture. Cook until the sauce begins to thicken, 1 to 2 minutes. Add the reserved tofu and toss to coat. Serve immediately.

Makes 4 servings.

JOSLIN CHOICES: 1 low-fat protein, 2 vegetable, 1 fat
PER SERVING: 162 calories (40% calories from fat), 8 g total fat (1 g saturated fat), 10 g protein,
   14 g carbohydrates, 3 g dietary fiber, 0 cholesterol, 378 mg sodium, 378 mg potassium

Tofu

Tofu is the "other white meat" for vegetarians. A good source of protein, tofu is low in calories and sodium and free of cholesterol. It is the product of soy milk, which is heated and mixed with coagulants to form the blocks. It has become widely available in both supermarkets and health food stores. Chinese-style tofu can be firm and chewy, while silken tofu will be custard-like. In our recipes calling for firm tofu, we suggest that you drain it well and press out any extra liquid before marinating it.

To press tofu, cut the block in half to form two thin rectangles. Place on one end of a kitchen towel or four-ply paper towels in a flat-bottomed bowl. Cover with waxed paper and more paper towels or the top of the kitchen towel. Weight it with a heavy pot or pan for 30 to 45 minutes at room temperature. Dry it off and you're ready to continue with the recipe. Getting the extra liquid out of the tofu will allow it to take on the tastes of your marinade without diluting the flavors.

Tofu should be fresh, so make sure to look at the date on the vacuum-packaged brand you purchase. It will keep three to four weeks in the refrigerator. Tofu is a chameleon, taking on the flavors of the closest sauce. Before cooking, it may be sliced and placed in a marinade for up to two days in your refrigerator. To freeze tofu, cut into slices, drain, wrap in plastic wrap, and place in a freezer bag. When ready to use, merely thaw and remove any liquid from the tofu.

Tofu enthusiasts use it for everything from burgers to shakes or even for mock cheese. You will find prepared tofu products in health food stores, as well as in your supermarket. These commercially made products make it easy to gain the benefit of eating this healthy soy product.

Vegetable Tofu Kebabs

Many people complain that tofu is bland. The answer to that problem is to marinate the tofu a long time or overnight. Be sure to first drain the tofu well and weight it down (see box above) so that any water in the tofu does not dilute the marinade.

12 ounces firm tofu, pressed and weighted, cut into cubes (see page 179)
2 tablespoons red wine vinegar
2 tablespoons reduced-sodium soy sauce
2 cloves garlic, pressed or minced
2 tablespoons olive oil
freshly ground pepper to taste
1 medium red bell pepper, seeded and cut into 8 squares
8 small button mushrooms
1 small yellow squash, cut into 8 slices
8 sweet onions, cut into 8 wedges

Place the tofu in a shallow dish. In a cup, whisk together the vinegar, soy sauce, garlic, oil, and pepper. Pour over the tofu and marinate for at least 1 hour, turning to coat each side.

Preheat the broiler.

Transfer the tofu to a paper towel to drain. Thread the tofu and vegetables onto 8 skewers and lightly brush the vegetables with the marinade. Broil, turning the kebabs, until the vegetables are done, about 2 to 3 minutes per side, turning 4 times.

Makes 4 servings.

JOSLIN CHOICES: 1 low-fat protein, 1 carbohydrate (bread/starch), 1 vegetable, 1 fat
PER SERVING: 216 calories (42% calories from fat), 11 g total fat (2 g saturated fat), 11 g protein,
    23 g carbohydrates, 4 g dietary fiber, 0 cholesterol, 287 mg sodium, 719 mg potassium

Vegetables

Golden Summer Frittata with Fresh Tomato Sauce

Come summer, we look for lighter fare, and this recipe makes the heat of the day take wing. At other times this makes a wonderful addition to a buffet brunch table and excels as the filling for a healthy cold sandwich.

2 large eggs
10 egg whites
2 tablespoons grated Parmesan cheese
¼ teaspoon salt (optional)
freshly ground pepper to taste
olive oil cooking spray
4 scallions, white part and 1 inch green, chopped
2 small zucchini, cut into 2-inch-long julienne strips
1 small yellow squash, cut into 2-inch-long julienne strips
1 small red bell pepper, seeded and cut into 2-inch-long julienne strips
1 tablespoon fresh thyme leaves
1 tablespoon finely chopped flat-leaf parsley
Fresh Tomato Sauce (recipe follows)

Preheat the broiler.

Whisk together the eggs and egg whites in a bowl with the Parmesan cheese, salt (if using), and pepper.

Lightly coat a nonstick skillet with an ovenproof handle with cooking spray. Add the scallions and sauté for 2 minutes. Add the zucchini, yellow squash, and bell pepper. Cook, stirring, until the vegetables are limp, about 5 minutes. Stir in the thyme and parsley.

Pour the eggs over the vegetables and cook over moderate heat, without stirring, for about 10 minutes, until the edges are beginning to brown and set. Place the frittata under the broiler and cook until puffed and brown, 4 to 5 minutes. Cut into 4 wedges and serve immediately with the Fresh Tomato Sauce.

Makes 4 servings.

JOSLIN CHOICES (WITH SAUCE): 2 low-fat protein, 1½ carbohydrate (bread/starch)
PER SERVING: 214 calories (21% calories from fat), 5 g total fat (2 g saturated fat), 19 g
    protein, 27 g carbohydrates, 6 g dietary fiber, 126 mg cholesterol, 416 mg sodium,
    1,366 mg potassium

Fresh Tomato Sauce

*T*his is a quick sauce to make when summer tomatoes are plentiful. Try it on pasta, as the sauce for a pizza, or with baked eggplant.

> *olive oil cooking spray*
> *1 small onion, minced*
> *3 pounds fresh tomatoes, peeled, seeded, and chopped*
> *¼ cup chopped fresh basil*
> *freshly ground pepper to taste*

Lightly coat a nonstick pot with cooking spray. Add the onion and sauté for 4 minutes, until soft. Add the tomatoes and cook for 15 to 20 minutes, stirring often, until the sauce thickens. Stir in the basil and pepper.

Makes about 2 cups.

JOSLIN CHOICES: 1 carbohydrate (bread/starch)

PER ½-CUP SERVING: 83 calories (11% calories from fat), 1 g total fat (0 saturated fat), 3 g protein, 18 g carbohydrates, 4 g dietary fiber, 0 cholesterol, 32 mg sodium, 812 mg potassium

Asparagus Flan

*T*his mild custard adds an elegant flare to any meal and can be made with other vegetables, such as broccoli, carrots, green beans, or squash.

> *1 pound thin asparagus, woody ends removed*
> *½ teaspoon minced garlic*
> *1 teaspoon minced fresh chives*
> *1 teaspoon minced fresh ginger*
> *⅛ teaspoon dry mustard*

⅓ cup plain nonfat yogurt
½ cup egg substitute
1 large egg white
⅛ teaspoon salt (optional)

Preheat the oven to 325°F.

Simmer the asparagus until tender, about 4 to 5 minutes. Drain and cut into 1-inch pieces, reserving 8 tips for garnish. Place the asparagus pieces in a food processor fitted with a metal blade. Add the garlic, chives, ginger, mustard, and yogurt. Process until the mixture becomes smooth. Add the egg substitute, egg white, and salt (if using). Process to combine well. Strain the mixture, using a wooden spoon to push through the sieve.

Place four ⅔-cup individual soufflé dishes in a baking pan. Fill each with ½ cup of the mixture. Fill the baking pan with hot water halfway up the sides of the soufflé dishes. Bake for about 40 minutes, until puffed and browned. Garnish with the reserved asparagus tips. Serve immediately.

Makes 4 servings.

JOSLIN CHOICES: I very-low-fat protein, I vegetable
PER SERVING: 68 calories (16% calories from fat), I g total fat (0 saturated fat), 8 g protein,
8 g carbohydrates, 2 g dietary fiber, I mg cholesterol, 160 mg sodium, 432 mg potassium

Broccoli, Italian-Style

*B*roccoli is a favorite vegetable in our home, and this is a particularly delicious way to prepare it. You'll find this dish served often throughout southern Italy, from the small family-style trattorias to the posh restaurants of Rome.

2 pounds fresh broccoli, broken into florets, stems peeled and chopped
2 teaspoons olive oil
12 large cloves garlic, peeled
1 small dried red chile pepper, crumbled

2 tablespoons dry white wine
salt to taste (optional)
freshly ground pepper to taste

Steam the broccoli over simmering water until tender and still bright green, about 10 minutes. Drain.

In a heavy nonstick skillet, heat the olive oil over medium heat. Add the garlic and chile pepper. Sauté for 2 minutes. Add the broccoli and wine; sauté, stirring, for 3 to 5 minutes.

Season with salt (if using) and pepper. Serve at once.

Makes 6 servings.

JOSLIN CHOICES: I vegetable
PER SERVING: 68 calories (23% calories from fat), 2 g total fat (0 saturated fat), 5 g protein,
10 g carbohydrates, 5 g dietary fiber, 0 cholesterol, 42 mg sodium, 522 mg potassium

Braised Celery

*O*ne doesn't often think of celery as a cooked vegetable, but prepared this way, it's absolutely delicious and so easy. You can cook the celery ahead of time and reheat to serve it hot, or serve it cold. Either way, it makes a welcome addition to almost any meal.

½ cup fresh lemon juice
2 teaspoons olive oil
1 pound (1 large bunch) celery, washed and sliced on the diagonal into 1-inch pieces
2 teaspoons ground cumin
⅛ teaspoon salt (optional)
freshly ground pepper to taste
minced flat-leaf parsley for garnish

In a large nonstick skillet, heat the lemon juice and olive oil. Add the celery, cumin, salt (if using), and pepper. Cover and simmer for 10 to 15 minutes, until tender but still crisp.

Remove from the heat and transfer to a serving bowl. Serve hot or chill to serve cold, sprinkled with the parsley.

Makes 4 servings.

JOSLIN CHOICES: 1 vegetable, ½ fat

PER SERVING: 52 calories (41% calories from fat), 3 g total fat (0 saturated fat), 1 g protein, 7 g carbohydrates, 2 g dietary fiber, 0 cholesterol, 101 mg sodium, 386 mg potassium

Baked Stuffed Chiles with Salsa

*R*emember that capsaicin, the ingredient in fresh chiles that inflames your taste buds, can do the same to your hands, eyes, and nose. So always wear rubber gloves when working with fresh chiles and immediately wash your hands thoroughly with soap and water after handling them.

6 large fresh poblano chiles

FRESH TOMATO SALSA
½ pound fresh ripe tomatoes, chopped
¼ cup finely minced onion
1 fresh jalapeño chile pepper, seeded and minced
½ tablespoon minced fresh cilantro
2 teaspoons fresh lemon juice
1 small clove garlic, minced
⅛ teaspoon salt (optional)

CHEESE FILLING
1 cup cooked white rice
½ cup shredded low-fat Monterey Jack cheese
¼ cup nonfat cottage cheese, drained
2 tablespoons minced red onion
1 tablespoon minced fresh cilantro

Preheat the broiler. Line a baking sheet with heavy-duty aluminum foil.

Rinse and dry the poblano chiles. Arrange on the prepared baking sheet. Broil until charred on all sides. Remove from the oven and wrap in the foil. Cool for 15 minutes. Set the oven temperature to 350°F.

Meanwhile, combine the salsa ingredients. Set aside.

When the chiles are cool enough to handle, peel them. Cut a lengthwise slit in each chile and carefully remove the seeds, keeping the stem intact.

To make the filling, in a medium bowl, combine the rice, ¼ cup shredded cheese, cottage cheese, red onion, and cilantro. Spoon the mixture into the chiles, closing the chiles to enclose the cheese mixture.

Spread half of the reserved salsa in the bottom of an 11 x 7-inch baking dish. Arrange the filled chiles on top of the salsa. Spoon the remaining salsa over the chiles and sprinkle with the remaining ¼ cup cheese. Bake until the cheese is melted and the chiles are heated through, about 15 to 20 minutes. Serve hot.

Makes 6 servings.

JOSLIN CHOICES: I carbohydrate (bread/starch)
PER SERVING: 99 calories (10% calories from fat), I g total fat (0 saturated fat), 6 g protein,
   17 g carbohydrates, I g dietary fiber, 3 mg cholesterol, 108 mg sodium, 246 mg potassium

Corn, Lima Bean, and Cucumber Succotash

*I*n the summer, use fresh corn and fresh lima beans in this sprightly version of an old-fashioned favorite vegetable. During the winter, frozen is just fine.

2 teaspoons canola oil
¼ cup minced white onion
1 cup lima beans
1 cup corn kernels
1 English (seedless) cucumber, peeled and coarsely chopped
½ cup diced red bell pepper
salt to taste (optional)
freshly ground pepper to taste

1 tablespoon fresh lemon juice
¼ cup minced fresh basil

In a large nonstick skillet, heat the oil over medium-low heat. Add the onion and sauté until limp but not browned, about 4 minutes.

Meanwhile, blanch the lima beans and corn in boiling water to cover for 3 minutes. Drain and set aside.

Add the cucumber and bell pepper to the skillet and sauté, stirring, until both are tender, about 6 minutes. Add the corn and lima beans and continue to cook, stirring occasionally, for another 2 to 3 minutes.

Taste and add salt (if using) and pepper. Drizzle with lemon juice and stir in the basil. Serve at once.

Makes 4 servings.

JOSLIN CHOICES: 1 carbohydrate (bread/starch)
PER SERVING: 119 calories (22% calories from fat), 3 g total fat (0 saturated fat), 5 g protein, 21 g carbohydrates, 4 g dietary fiber, 0 cholesterol, 7 mg sodium, 438 mg potassium

Curried Cauliflower, Peas, and Potatoes

*I*ndian cooks have a glorious way with vegetables, and this recipe is a prime example. The mélange of aromas will make calling your family for dinner a second time a thing of the past. Available in Indian and Asian markets, garam masala is a blend of dry-roasted spices from northern India. You can make your own following the recipe on page 86.

2 small thin-skinned potatoes, scrubbed and cut into 1-inch cubes
vegetable cooking spray
1 teaspoon ground cumin
4½ tablespoons minced fresh ginger
¼ teaspoon cayenne pepper
4 teaspoons ground coriander
1 teaspoon turmeric
1 large onion, diced

1 small head cauliflower (about ¾ pound), cut into bite-size pieces, florets and tender stems only
⅔ cup water
1 10-ounce package frozen baby peas, unthawed
1 teaspoon garam masala (page 86)
¼ teaspoon salt (optional)

Simmer the potatoes in salted water until they are cooked through when tested with the tip of a knife, about 5 to 6 minutes. Drain and set aside.

Lightly coat a nonstick pot with cooking spray and heat until hot. Toast the cumin, stirring, for 20 seconds. Add the ginger, cayenne, coriander, and turmeric. Cook for 30 seconds more. Add the onion and cook over medium-low heat until transparent and limp, about 3 to 4 minutes. Stir in the cauliflower and turn to coat with the spices. Add the water, cover, and simmer until the vegetables are cooked, 8 to 10 minutes. Add the peas and potatoes and cook a few minutes more, until heated through.

Just before serving, stir in the garam masala and salt (if using). Serve immediately.

Makes 4 servings.

JOSLIN CHOICES: 1½ carbohydrate (bread/starch)
PER SERVING: 140 calories (5% calories from fat), 1 g total fat (0 saturated fat), 5 g protein,
    29 g carbohydrates, 6 g dietary fiber, 0 cholesterol, 396 mg sodium, 543 mg potassium

Eggplant and Tomato Tart

This elegant tart is easy enough to make whenever you feel like pampering yourself or guests. Feel free to substitute zucchini or summer squash for the eggplant or red bell pepper for the tomato. For extra zip, use sweet onion slices when available.

butter-flavored cooking spray
1 medium eggplant, cut into ¼-inch-thick rounds
6 sheets filo pastry

1 cup egg substitute

4 ounces low-fat feta cheese, crumbled

2 cloves garlic, minced

¼ cup chopped fresh basil

1 large tomato, thinly sliced

Preheat the oven to 425°F. Lightly coat a nonstick baking sheet with cooking spray.

Place the eggplant slices on the prepared sheet. Lightly coat the eggplant with more of the cooking spray and bake until soft, about 20 minutes, turning once.

While the eggplant is baking, place 1 sheet of filo in an 11-inch tart pan. Lightly coat with cooking spray. Repeat with 5 more filo layers, spraying between each layer. Cut any overhang, leaving 1 inch. Turn the edge over and crimp. Lightly coat with cooking spray.

In a small bowl, combine the egg substitute, cheese, garlic, and basil. Pour into the pastry-lined pan. Top with the cooked eggplant and sliced tomato. Bake for 35 to 40 minutes, until the filling is cooked and the filo is browned. Serve immediately.

Makes 4 servings.

JOSLIN CHOICES: 3 low-fat protein, 1½ carbohydrate (bread/starch)

PER SERVING: 300 calories (31% calories from fat), 10 g total fat (4 g saturated fat), 24 g protein, 28 g carbohydrates, 5 g dietary fiber, 11 mg cholesterol, 743 mg sodium, 852 mg potassium

Stuffed Eggplant

*W*hen we think of comfort food, this dish is high on our list. Serve it as the main course or in smaller portions with an herbed omelet.

olive oil cooking spray

2 eggplants (about ¾ pound each)

1 medium onion, minced

¼ pound button mushrooms, chopped

1 large clove garlic, minced

1 small red bell pepper, seeded and chopped
1 cup cooked rice
1 teaspoon finely chopped fresh thyme
1 teaspoon finely chopped fresh marjoram
2 teaspoons finely chopped fresh oregano
⅛ teaspoon salt (optional)
freshly ground pepper to taste
2 tablespoons grated Romano cheese
1 14½-ounce can no-salt-added diced tomatoes

Preheat the oven to 350°F. Lightly coat a large baking dish with cooking spray.

Place the eggplants in a large kettle of boiling water and simmer, covered, for 15 minutes. Drain and cut in half lengthwise. Carefully remove the pulp, leaving a shell ½ inch thick. Chop the pulp and set aside.

Coat a nonstick skillet with cooking spray and sauté the onion, mushrooms, garlic, and bell pepper until just tender. Add the reserved eggplant, rice, thyme, marjoram, oregano, salt (if using), and pepper. Cook for 2 minutes. Remove from the heat and stir in the Romano cheese.

Stuff the eggplant shells with the vegetable mixture and place in the prepared baking dish. Pour the tomatoes on top of the eggplant. Bake for 20 to 25 minutes, until heated through. Serve immediately.

Makes 4 servings.

JOSLIN CHOICES: 2 carbohydrate (bread/starch)
PER SERVING: 164 calories (8% calories from fat), 2 g total fat (1 g saturated fat), 6 g protein, 34 g carbohydrates, 7 g dietary fiber, 3 mg cholesterol, 127 mg sodium, 826 mg potassium

Vegetable Moussaka

*N*othing fills the kitchen with the heavenly aroma of exotic spice combinations more than moussaka with cinnamon, cumin, and mint. Here we use brown rice, but you might try a fragrant rice such as basmati for a change. Add a dollop of the yogurt-based sauce, and you have a sensational moussaka that should put the dish frequently on your menu.

> *olive oil cooking spray*
> *1 large eggplant, cut into ¼-inch-thick rounds*
> *1 onion, chopped*
> *1 tablespoon slivered almonds*
> *1 28-ounce can no-salt-added crushed tomatoes*
> *¼ cup dried currants*
> *1 teaspoon ground cinnamon*
> *1 teaspoon ground cumin*
> *¼ cup packed chopped fresh mint*
> *2 teaspoons fresh lemon juice*
> *freshly ground pepper to taste*
> *2½ cups cooked brown rice*

> YOGURT SAUCE
> *1 cup plain nonfat yogurt*
> *3 tablespoons chopped fresh mint*
> *⅛ teaspoon salt (optional)*
> *freshly ground pepper to taste*
> *½ teaspoon grated lemon zest*

Preheat the oven to 375°F. Lightly coat a large nonstick baking sheet with cooking spray.

Place the eggplant slices on the prepared baking sheet. Lightly coat the eggplant with more of the cooking spray and bake until soft, about 20 minutes, turning once.

While the eggplant is baking, coat a large nonstick saucepan with cooking spray. Add the onion and almonds; sauté for 3 minutes, until the onion is soft. Add the tomatoes, currants, cinnamon, cumin, mint, and lemon juice. Simmer for 5 minutes. Season with pepper and stir in the rice. Set aside.

Prepare the sauce by combining the yogurt, mint, salt (if using), pepper, and lemon zest. Refrigerate until ready to serve.

Line the bottom and sides of a 9-inch square baking dish with half of the cooked eggplant slices. Fill with the tomato-rice mixture. Top with the remaining eggplant slices. Cover with aluminum foil and bake for 1 hour on a baking sheet to protect your oven from spills. Remove from the oven and allow to rest for 15 minutes. To serve, cut into squares and top with a dollop of yogurt sauce.

Makes 8 servings.

JOSLIN CHOICES: 1½ carbohydrate (bread/starch)
PER SERVING: 135 calories (9% calories from fat), 1 g total fat (0 saturated fat), 5 g protein,
  28 g carbohydrates, 5 g dietary fiber, 1 mg cholesterol, 70 mg sodium, 460 mg potassium

Green Beans with Pistachios

This simple, colorful vegetable accompaniment goes with many entrées. When fresh asparagus is in season, substitute it for the green beans. If you don't have pistachios, used sliced almonds.

> *1 pound green beans, trimmed*
> *butter-flavored cooking spray*
> *2 shallots, minced*
> *1 large tomato, seeded and chopped*
> *1 tablespoon chopped flat-leaf parsley*
> *1 teaspoon fresh lemon juice*
> *salt to taste (optional)*
> *freshly ground pepper to taste*
> *2 tablespoons chopped pistachios*

Cook the green beans in boiling water to cover until crisp-tender, about 3 to 4 minutes. Drain and keep warm.

Lightly coat a large nonstick skillet with cooking spray. Add the shallots and sauté over medium-low heat, stirring occasionally, until limp, about 5 minutes. Add the tomato, parsley, lemon juice, salt (if using), and pepper. Cook until heated through, about 2 minutes.

Place the green beans in a serving dish. Spoon the tomato mixture over the beans and sprinkle with pistachios. Serve at once.

Makes 4 servings.

JOSLIN CHOICES: I vegetable, I fat
PER SERVING: 90 calories (33% calories from fat), 4 g total fat (0 saturated fat), 4 g protein, 13 g carbohydrates, 5 g dietary fiber, 0 cholesterol, 12 mg sodium, 440 mg potassium

Leeks and Peppers, Italian-Style

This colorful mélange is best in the summer when fresh local leeks are available, but try it with scallions or mild onions throughout the year. Serve it with your favorite grain pilaf, such as kasha, couscous, or brown rice, or for a change add cooked potatoes to the leek and pepper combination.

4 large leeks, trimmed
1 tablespoon olive oil
2 medium yellow bell peppers, seeded and cut into thin strips
2 medium red bell peppers, seeded and cut into thin strips
⅓ cup chopped fresh basil or flat-leaf parsley
freshly ground pepper to taste
butter-flavored cooking spray

Cut the leeks in half and wash well between each layer. Cut into thin half-circle slices and set aside.

Heat the oil in a large nonstick skillet. Add the leeks, cover, and cook, stirring once, for 3 minutes. Add the bell peppers, cover, and simmer until all the vegetables are soft, an additional 5 minutes. Add the basil or parsley and pepper. Cook for another minute. Lightly coat with cooking spray just before you serve.

Makes 6 servings.

JOSLIN CHOICES: I carbohydrate (bread/starch)

PER SERVING: 84 calories (26% calories from fat), 3 g total fat (0 saturated fat), 2 g protein, 15 g carbohydrates, 3 g dietary fiber, 0 cholesterol, 14 mg sodium, 320 mg potassium

Baked Potato and Squash Casserole

This robust casserole is truly splendid and redolent of Italian flavor. Feel free to add tomatoes if you like and to substitute fresh oregano for the parsley.

olive oil cooking spray
1¼ pounds russet potatoes, scrubbed and cut into 1½-inch pieces
2 yellow squash, cut into 1½-inch pieces
2 zucchini, cut into 1½-inch pieces
½ red bell pepper, cut into 1-inch pieces
3 cloves garlic, minced
2 teaspoons paprika
⅓ cup chopped flat-leaf parsley
1 tablespoon balsamic vinegar
1 tablespoon olive oil
⅛ teaspoon salt (optional)
freshly ground pepper to taste
1 tablespoon freshly grated Parmesan cheese

Preheat the oven to 375°F. Lightly coat a baking dish big enough for the vegetables with cooking spray.

Boil the potatoes in lightly salted water until just tender, about 10 minutes. Drain and place in the baking dish. Add the squash, zucchini, bell pepper, and garlic. Mix well. Toss with the paprika and parsley. Sprinkle with the vinegar, oil, salt (if using), and pepper. Toss once again to coat.

Cover the dish with aluminum foil and bake for 35 to 40 minutes. Uncover, lightly coat the top with cooking spray, sprinkle with the Parmesan cheese, and bake for another 15 minutes, until the vegetables are browned. Serve immediately.

Makes 6 servings.

JOSLIN CHOICES: I carbohydrate (bread/starch), I vegetable

PER SERVING: 138 calories (19% calories from fat), 3 g total fat (1 g saturated fat), 5 g protein, 26 g carbohydrates, 5 g dietary fiber, I mg cholesterol, 80 mg sodium, 791 mg potassium

Potatoes: They Come in All Sizes and Colors

Considering their lowly heritage as peasant food for centuries, potatoes have today become fashionable. They come in a variety of sizes, from the tiny new potatoes about I inch in diameter, called creamers, to large russets that weigh almost a pound. One of our favorite comfort foods, potatoes also come in a variety of colors. Look for these in the gourmet produce section of your supermarket, at farmer's markets, and at natural foods stores:

All red: a midseason potato with bright red skin and reddish, waxy flesh

Butterfinger: a mid- to late-season fingerling variety with a yellow, buttery flesh

Candy-strips: an unusual midseason variety with red strips running through its white flesh

Caribe: an early season potato with blue skin and a light, starchy white flesh

French fingerling: a tasty fingerling with purple skin and yellow flesh

Katahdin: a northeastern late-season variety with brown skin and white, starchy flesh

Lehmi russet: a very large, late-season potato with brown skin and white flesh

Ruby crescent: flavor-packed, mid- to late-season variety with rosy-colored skin and yellow, waxy flesh

Yukon Gold: a small, early-season variety with yellow skin and flesh and a distinctive buttery flavor

Roasted Potatoes, Portuguese-Style

*W*e've always been intrigued by the lively, spicy flavors of Portuguese food. Here we've adapted a native dish using coriander, a spice the Portuguese often use with potatoes.

olive oil cooking spray
6 5-ounce Yukon Gold or russet potatoes, scrubbed
2 tablespoons olive oil
2 teaspoons ground coriander
2 tablespoons chopped fresh cilantro
1 tablespoon sliced almonds

Preheat the oven to 350°F. Lightly coat a large nonstick baking sheet with cooking spray.

Slice the potatoes into rounds about ½ inch thick. Place in a large bowl and drizzle with the olive oil. Mix to coat evenly. Arrange the potatoes in a single layer on the prepared baking sheet.

Roast until tender, about 45 minutes, turning once after 30 minutes. Transfer the potatoes to a serving bowl. Sprinkle with the coriander, cilantro, and almonds. Toss and serve.

Makes 6 servings.

JOSLIN CHOICES: 1½ carbohydrate (bread/starch), 1 fat
PER SERVING: 143 calories (32% calories from fat), 5 g total fat (1 g saturated fat), 3 g protein, 22 g carbohydrates, 2 g dietary fiber, 0 cholesterol, 8 mg sodium, 679 mg potassium

Acorn Squash with Garlic Custard and Wild Mushrooms

*T*his recipe is inspired by a dish that we've enjoyed over and over at our friend Carole Peck's Good News Café in Woodbury, Connecticut. Carol makes this using whole baby pumpkins, which are available only for a very short time in the early fall. Since we like the combination so much, we've tried using acorn squash with excellent results. The garlic custard—from our earlier cookbook, *The Joslin Diabetes Gourmet Cookbook*—is our lightened version of the garlic custard made famous by cookbook author Paula Wolfert.

The recipe may seem daunting at first glance, but since both the custard and squash bake in the same oven while you sauté the mushrooms, the dish actually goes together quite easily and is well worth the effort. Each bite offers the savory flavor of the squash, the piquancy of the garlic custard, and the exotic taste of wild mushrooms. If you find it hard to cut an acorn squash, ask your produce person to do it for you. Most will gladly do so—without any charge.

Try the garlic custard as a side dish with any meal—it's an excellent addition to almost any dinner.

olive oil cooking spray

GARLIC CUSTARD
10 cloves garlic, roasted
1½ cups evaporated skim milk
2 large eggs
2 teaspoons fresh thyme leaves or ½ teaspoon crushed dried
freshly ground pepper to taste

ACORN SQUASH AND WILD MUSHROOMS
1 large acorn squash (about 2 pounds)
salt to taste (optional)
1 tablespoon olive oil
1¼ pounds mixed fresh mushrooms (such as porcini, shiitake, chanterelle, or button),
*   thinly sliced*
2 tablespoons fresh lemon juice
freshly ground pepper to taste

Preheat the oven to 350°F. Lightly spray six ½-cup custard cups with cooking spray. Set in a medium baking pan with at least 2-inch sides.

To make the garlic custard, peel and squeeze the garlic cloves into a food processor or blender. Add the milk and process until smooth. Add the eggs, thyme, and pepper and process again. Divide the mixture among the prepared custard cups.

To prepare the squash, cut it in half, then cut each half into 3 wedges. Do not peel. Using a spoon, scrape out the seeds and fibers. Place the squash wedges cut side down in a large baking pan and add about 2 inches of water and the salt (if using).

Pour boiling water into the baking pan with the custard to come halfway up the sides of the cups. Bake the custard and squash in the oven at the same time. Bake the squash for 30 to 35 minutes, until tender when pierced with a fork. Bake the custard until gently set, about 35 minutes. Remove and set the cups on a rack for 5 minutes.

While the custard and squash are baking, heat the oil in a large nonstick skillet over medium-high heat. Add the mushrooms and sauté, stirring occasionally, until tender and almost all of the liquid is evaporated, about 8 to 10 minutes. Add the lemon juice, salt (if using), and pepper; stir and cook for another minute. Remove from the heat and keep warm.

To serve, arrange a wedge of squash, peel side down, on a large plate. Run a thin-bladed knife around the outer edge of each custard cup and unmold a custard into the center of each squash wedge. Distribute the warm mushrooms over and around the garlic custards. Serve at once.

Makes 6 servings.

JOSLIN CHOICES: ½ low-fat protein, 2 carbohydrate (bread/starch)

PER SERVING: 188 calories (21% calories from fat), 5 g total fat (1 g saturated fat), 10 g protein, 30 g carbohydrates, 3 g dietary fiber, 73 mg cholesterol, 152 mg sodium, 1,136 mg potassium

JOSLIN CHOICES (garlic custard only): ½ carbohydrate (nonfat milk)

PER SERVING: 83 calories (24% calories from fat), 2 g total fat (1 g saturated fat), 7 g protein, 9 g carbohydrates, 0 dietary fiber, 73 mg cholesterol, 96 mg sodium, 255 mg potassium

Oven-Roasted Butternut Squash with Onions, Chestnuts, and Apples

Oven-roasting caramelizes the natural sugars in vegetables, making them taste and smell wonderful. Fresh chestnuts, which are very low in fat, add a distinctive flavor to the mix. If fresh chestnuts aren't available, you can purchase them already roasted and shelled in a jar.

½ pound fresh chestnuts
½ pound pearl onions
butter-flavored cooking spray
1 teaspoon reduced-fat margarine
1 teaspoon canola oil
1½ pounds butternut squash, peeled and cut into ½-inch cubes
salt to taste (optional)
freshly ground pepper to taste
1 cup canned low-fat, low-sodium chicken or vegetable broth
1 teaspoon minced fresh thyme or ¼ teaspoon crushed dried
1 large Granny Smith or other tart cooking apple, peeled, cored, and cut into ½-inch
*   cubes*
½ cup unsweetened apple juice

Using a sharp knife, make an X on the flat side of each chestnut. Place in a medium saucepan and cover with water. Place over medium heat and bring to a boil. Reduce the heat and simmer for 20 to 30 minutes. Drain and allow to cool slightly, then peel off the shells and inner skins. Break the peeled nuts into ½-inch pieces. Set aside.

Refill the saucepan with fresh water and bring to a rapid boil. Add the pearl onions and cook for 4 minutes. Drain, rinse, and drain again. With a sharp knife, trim off the root end from each onion and slip off the skin.

Preheat the oven to 450°F. Lightly coat a large roasting pan with cooking spray. Add the margarine and oil and place in the oven for 3 minutes.

Spread the onions and butternut squash in the roasting pan; season with salt (if using) and pepper. Roast the vegetables for 25 minutes, stirring occasionally, until tender and browned.

Meanwhile, combine the peeled chestnuts, broth, and thyme in a medium saucepan. Bring to a boil over high heat and cook until the liquid is reduced by two-thirds, about 5 minutes.

Sprinkle the apples over the roasted vegetables and stir in the apple juice. Continue to roast for another 5 minutes. Transfer the roasted vegetables and apples to a large serving bowl and stir in the chestnut-broth mixture. Serve at once.

Makes 6 servings.

JOSLIN CHOICES: 2 carbohydrate (bread/starch)
PER SERVING: 185 calories (10% calories from fat), 2 g total fat (0 saturated fat), 3 g protein,
41 g carbohydrates, 8 g dietary fiber, 1 mg cholesterol, 87 mg sodium, 634 mg potassium

Spinach Roulade

*T*his elegant rolled soufflé will astound your guests and make your family feel really special—and no one need ever know how easy it was to make. You can substitute nonfat ricotta cheese for the cottage cheese with excellent results, and finely minced broccoli for the spinach.

> *butter-flavored cooking spray*
> *2 teaspoons reduced-fat margarine*
> *2 tablespoons finely grated Parmesan cheese*
> *2 scallions, minced*
> *1 10-ounce package frozen chopped spinach, thawed*
> *½ cup plus 2 tablespoons egg substitute*
> *⅛ teaspoon ground nutmeg*
> *⅛ teaspoon salt (optional)*
> *freshly ground pepper to taste*
> *5 large egg whites*
> *1 cup nonfat cottage cheese, drained*
> *⅛ teaspoon garlic powder*
> *2 tablespoons chopped flat-leaf parsley*
> *2 tablespoons chopped fresh basil*
> *chopped tomatoes for garnish*

Preheat the oven to 375°F.

Coat a 15 x 10¼-inch jelly roll pan with cooking spray and line with aluminum foil. Grease the foil with margarine and sprinkle with 1 tablespoon Parmesan cheese. Set aside.

Lightly coat a small nonstick skillet with cooking spray. Add the scallions and sauté for 1 minute. Squeeze all the liquid from the spinach and add to the skillet, breaking it up with a wooden spoon. Remove from the heat. Stir in the egg substitute, nutmeg, salt (if using), and pepper.

Beat the egg whites until stiff but not dry. Gently stir one-quarter of the beaten egg whites into the spinach mixture. Carefully fold in the remaining beaten egg whites. Spoon the soufflé mixture into the prepared pan, using a spatula to smooth the top and fill the corners. Bake about 20 minutes, until puffed and golden brown.

Place the cottage cheese in a food processor fitted with a metal blade. Add the garlic powder and blend until smooth and creamy. Add the chopped herbs and ground pepper. Set aside.

When the soufflé is done, turn out onto a piece of waxed paper sprinkled with the remaining tablespoon of Parmesan cheese. Carefully remove the aluminum foil. When cool, spread the top with the cottage cheese mixture. Tightly roll the roulade from one of the long sides, either toward or away from you (whichever seems easier). Roll the paper tightly around the roulade and chill. Serve cold, or warm in a 375°F oven for 8 to 10 minutes. Slice into 1-inch rounds with a sharp serrated knife. Garnish with chopped tomatoes.

Makes 6 servings.

JOSLIN CHOICES: 1½ very-low-fat protein, 1 vegetable
PER SERVING: 91 calories (24% calories from fat), 2 g total fat (1 g saturated fat),
   3 g protein, 4 g carbohydrates, 1 g dietary fiber, 5 mg cholesterol, 346 mg sodium,
   279 mg potassium

Whipped Sweet Potatoes

*H*ere's a recipe for really good, fluffy sweet potatoes. Since it's so easy to prepare, keep it in mind throughout the fall and winter months, not just for holiday meals.

1½ pounds sweet potatoes, peeled and cut into 1-inch pieces
2 medium carrots (about ½ pound), peeled and cut into 1-inch pieces
¼ cup evaporated skim milk

1½ tablespoons reduced-fat margarine
½ teaspoon salt (optional)
1 tablespoon brown sugar
2 tablespoons fresh orange juice
⅛ teaspoon ground nutmeg

Place the sweet potatoes and carrots in a large saucepan with cold water to cover. Bring to a boil, reduce the heat, and simmer until the vegetables are very tender, about 15 to 20 minutes. Drain.

Return the vegetables to the pan. Add the milk, margarine, salt (if using), brown sugar, orange juice, and nutmeg. Mash the potato mixture over low heat, then whip the potatoes to the desired consistency. Serve immediately.

Makes 6 servings.

JOSLIN CHOICES: 2 carbohydrate (bread/starch)
PER SERVING: 140 calories (14% calories from fat), 2 g total fat (0 saturated fat), 3 g protein, 28 g carbohydrates, 2 g dietary fiber, 1 mg cholesterol, 58 mg sodium, 452 mg potassium

Slow-Roasted Plum Tomatoes

This is one of our favorite ways to prepare tomatoes in the dead of winter, when the only decent tomatoes in the supermarket are the Roma (plum) variety or imported tomatoes that sell for an exorbitant price. Just a sprinkling of sugar brings out the plum tomatoes' natural sweetness as they dry during a long, slow roasting. Serve these with any grilled fish, meat, or fowl. They are also delicious spread over grilled or toasted peasant bread.

8 ripe plum tomatoes (about 1¼ pounds)
1 tablespoon olive oil
1 teaspoon sugar
salt to taste (optional)
freshly ground pepper to taste
1 tablespoon fresh thyme leaves or 1 teaspoon crushed dried

1 teaspoon chopped fresh rosemary or ¼ teaspoon crushed dried

Preheat the oven to 250°F. Line a baking sheet with parchment paper or aluminum foil.

Arrange the tomatoes on the prepared baking sheet and brush the tops with olive oil. Sprinkle with the sugar, salt (if using), pepper, 2 teaspoons of the fresh thyme leaves (or ¾ teaspoon dried), and the rosemary.

Bake until reduced in size and velvety soft, about 1½ to 2 hours.

Using a spatula, carefully transfer the tomatoes to a serving platter and sprinkle with the remaining thyme. Serve at once.

Makes 4 servings.

JOSLIN CHOICES: 1 vegetable, 1 fat
PER SERVING: 63 calories (49% calories from fat), 4 g total fat (1 g saturated fat), 1 g protein,
   7 g carbohydrates, 2 g dietary fiber, 0 cholesterol, 12 mg sodium, 279 mg potassium

Spaghetti Squash with Savory Ratatouille

We love to make this when fresh basil, fresh ripe tomatoes, and tender zucchini are at their seasonal peak, but we do admit to also making it in the dead of winter using canned no-salt-added tomatoes and dried basil. It's so colorful and delicious it's sure to become a family favorite.

1 spaghetti squash (about 2 pounds)
1 small eggplant (about ¾ pound), cut in half lengthwise
1 tablespoon olive oil
2 medium onions, sliced
4 cloves garlic, chopped
1 large red bell pepper, seeded, cut in half crosswise, then cut into ½-inch-wide strips
1 large green bell pepper, seeded, cut in half crosswise, then cut into ½-inch-wide strips
4 medium ripe tomatoes, peeled, seeded, and coarsely chopped
1 small bay leaf

½ teaspoon crushed dried oregano
¼ teaspoon crushed dried thyme
salt to taste (optional)
freshly ground pepper to taste
¾ pound small zucchini, stems trimmed and thickly sliced
3 tablespoons chopped fresh basil or 1 teaspoon crushed dried
⅛ teaspoon cayenne pepper
chopped flat-leaf parsley for garnish (optional)

Preheat the oven to 350°F. Pierce the spaghetti squash deeply 2 or 3 times with a sharp carving fork to keep it from exploding. Place on a baking sheet and bake until tender when pierced with a knife, about 1½ hours.

Meanwhile, score the eggplant down the center of the cut sides, being careful not to cut through to the skin. Place cut side down on a baking sheet and bake for 30 minutes, until the skin begins to shrivel. Remove from the oven and allow to cool. Dice and set aside.

In a large heavy saucepan, heat the oil over medium heat. Add the onions, garlic, and bell peppers. Cook, stirring occasionally, until the vegetables are limp, about 5 minutes. Add the tomatoes, reserved eggplant, bay leaf, and dried herbs. Cover partially and simmer over low heat for 45 minutes, stirring occasionally. Taste and add salt (if using) and pepper.

Stir in the zucchini and continue to cook, partially covered, for 5 minutes. Stir in the basil and cayenne. Remove the bay leaf.

When the spaghetti squash is done, remove it from the oven and cut in half. Scoop out the seeds. Comb the strands of squash pulp out of each half with 2 forks and place on a large round platter. Pile the eggplant-tomato mixture in the center and garnish with chopped parsley. Serve hot.

Makes 4 servings.

JOSLIN CHOICES: 2 carbohydrate (bread/starch), 1 fat
PER SERVING: 228 calories (21% calories from fat), 6 g total fat (1 g saturated fat), 8 g
    protein, 43 g carbohydrates, 11 g dietary fiber, 0 cholesterol, 64 mg sodium, 1,483 mg
    potassium

Zucchini Lasagna

*W*hen is zucchini not just another green vegetable? When it stands in for pasta. Here we slice this year-round favorite lengthwise into pasta-thin slices and layer it with cheeses and other vegetables to make a lasagna that will become one of your favorites. Like its high-calorie cousin, this one is also great reheated or even cold for lunch the next day.

1½ pounds small zucchini, ends removed, washed, and cut lengthwise into thin slices
salt

SAUCE
olive oil cooking spray
1 small onion, minced
3 cloves garlic, minced
1 6-ounce container sliced Italian cremini mushrooms
1 28-ounce can no-salt-added crushed tomatoes
½ teaspoon crushed fennel seeds
2 sprigs oregano
freshly ground pepper to taste

CHEESE FILLING
1 15-ounce container fat-free ricotta cheese
1 small carrot, grated
1 10-ounce package frozen chopped spinach, thawed, all liquid squeezed out
¼ cup egg substitute
1 cup grated low-fat mozzarella cheese
2 tablespoons grated Parmesan cheese
⅓ cup chopped fresh basil
freshly ground pepper to taste

Preheat the oven to 400°F.

Lightly salt the zucchini slices on both sides and allow to weep for 20 minutes. Carefully wipe off all salt and liquid and set aside.

To make the sauce, coat a large nonstick pot with cooking spray and add the onion. Cook for 2 minutes over medium heat, until the onion begins to soften. Add the garlic and mushrooms and cook an additional 2 minutes. Stir in the tomatoes, fennel seeds, oregano, and pepper. Simmer while you continue to prepare the recipe.

To make the filling, place the ricotta in a bowl and stir in the carrot, spinach, egg substitute, mozzarella cheese, 1 tablespoon Parmesan cheese, basil, and pepper. Combine well and set aside.

Remove the oregano sprigs from the sauce. Coat the bottom of a 9-inch square baking pan with 3 tablespoons of sauce. Layer the bottom with slices of zucchini.

Spread half of the cheese mixture on top and then ladle half of the tomato sauce over all. Repeat the process, ending with sauce. Place the pan on a baking sheet and cover with aluminum foil. Bake for 45 minutes.

Remove the foil, top with the remaining Parmesan cheese, and bake, uncovered, for 15 minutes longer, until the lasagna is bubbling and the cheese is melted. Remove from the oven and allow to rest for 15 minutes before serving.

Makes 6 servings.

JOSLIN CHOICES: 2½ low-fat protein, 1 carbohydrate (bread/starch)

PER SERVING: 242 calories (36% calories from fat), 10 g total fat (6 g saturated fat), 20 g protein, 20 g carbohydrates, 5 g dietary fiber, 34 mg cholesterol, 352 mg sodium, 1,081 mg potassium

FRUITS AND OTHER SWEETS

Apricot and Orange Fool

You can use any stewed and pureed fruit to make a fool, and for a change you can add any orange-flavored liqueur to the recipe to add to its delicacy. If you grow rhubarb, you can use the recipe with ground ginger for another delicious version.

Uncooked egg whites are no longer considered safe by the United States Department of Agriculture, since raw eggs have been found to be a possible carrier of food-borne illness. This recipe calls for pasteurized egg whites, which are easy to measure, whip up exactly like raw egg whites, and eliminate the possibility of any contamination. You'll find the product in the dairy section of your supermarket, usually next to the egg substitute.

> 1 6-ounce package dried apricots
> 1½ cups plain nonfat yogurt
> 1 to 2 packets sugar substitute, depending on taste
> ¼ cup pasteurized liquid egg whites
> grated zest of ½ orange
> mint leaves for garnish

Cover the apricots with water and simmer over low heat for 20 minutes, until very soft. Place the yogurt in a paper-lined strainer to drain while the apricots are simmering.

Drain the apricots and puree in a food processor fitted with a metal blade. Combine the puree with the drained yogurt and sugar substitute. Beat the egg whites until they form peaks. Add a dollop to the puree to loosen it, then fold in the remainder. Fold in the orange zest.

Place the fool in decorative glass dessert cups and serve garnished with mint.

Makes 4 servings.

JOSLIN CHOICES: I very-low-fat protein, 2 carbohydrate (fruit)

PER SERVING: 161 calories (1% calories from fat), 0 total fat, 0 saturated fat, 7 g protein, 35 g carbohydrates, 2 g dietary fiber, 2 mg cholesterol, 77 mg sodium, 578 mg potassium

Bananas Havana

*I*t used to be that only one kind of bananas was sold at the supermarket, but recently we've been seeing imports from South America and the Caribbean with exotic names. If your market has them, substitute one of the "new" bananas for the more common variety.

3 large ripe, firm bananas, cut in half crosswise
1 fresh lime, quartered
butter-flavored cooking spray
1 tablespoon reduced-fat margarine
2 tablespoons light brown sugar
3 tablespoons rum (optional)
1 tablespoon sliced almonds

Peel the bananas and cut in half lengthwise. Squeeze lime juice over each banana quarter.

Lightly coat a large nonstick skillet with cooking spray. Add the margarine and place over medium heat. Add the bananas and sauté for 2 minutes per side, turning once. Sprinkle the bananas with brown sugar; sauté for 1 minute more.

Remove from the heat and pour on the rum (if using). Carefully ignite the rum and shake the skillet until the flames are extinguished. Sprinkle with the almonds and serve 2 quarters per person on individual dessert plates.

Makes 6 servings.

JOSLIN CHOICES: 1½ carbohydrate (fruit)

PER SERVING: 115 calories (16% calories from fat), 2 g total fat (0 saturated fat), 1 g protein, 22 g carbohydrates, 2 g dietary fiber, 0 cholesterol, 22 mg sodium, 304 mg potassium

Artificial Sweeteners

Although nutrition guidelines no longer view eating sugar as unsafe for people with diabetes, it must be counted as part of your allotment of carbohydrates. Be aware that many foods that have sugar often have a high fat content. These foods should be used only on special occasions.

Artificial sweeteners (noncaloric), on the other hand, are "free foods" and therefore do not raise blood glucose levels and can be added to a meal plan. Moderate amounts of these sweeteners can be used to make many of the special things that people with diabetes may feel they have missed.

Saccharin: Saccharin, which is 200 to 700 times sweeter than table sugar, can be used to sweeten either hot or cold foods. Pregnant women are cautioned not to use it. You can purchase saccharin under the brand names of Sucaryl, Sugar Twin, Sweet Magic, Sweet'n Low, and Zero-Cal.

Aspartame: This sweetener is 160 to 220 times sweeter than table sugar and is not appropriate for recipes that are cooked more than 20 minutes, as the chemical compound breaks down. It is therefore suggested that it be added at the very end of cooking recipes like puddings. People with a rare condition called phenylketonuria (PKU) should avoid aspartame. Otherwise, it is a safe sweetener. The brand names are Equal, Sweetmate, and Spoonfuls.

Acesulfame Potassium: This sweetener, also known as acesulfame-K, came on the market in 1988. It can be used in baking and cooking because it does not break down when heated. Two hundred times sweeter than table sugar, it is often used with sugar in baking to achieve the desired texture. The tabletop sweetener is called Sweet One.

Sucralose: This product, which is made from sucrose, was approved in 1998 and is 600 times sweeter than table sugar. It can be used in recipes that require prolonged heating without losing any of its sweetness. It has no reported side effects or restrictions on its use by pregnant women. It can be purchased under the brand name Splenda at your supermarket.

Poached Pears with Almond Cream

We always used to peel pears before poaching. What a wonderful discovery when we skipped the peeling and cooked them with the skin intact. The rustic appearance is very appealing.

> *4 small firm Bosc pears (about 1 pound total)*
> *1½ cups dry white wine or unsweetened apple juice*
> *1¾ cups water*
> *3 whole peppercorns*
> *2 whole cloves*
> *1 3-inch cinnamon stick*

> ALMOND CREAM
> *½ cup fat-free sour cream*
> *1 tablespoon light brown sugar*
> *½ tablespoon almond-flavored liqueur or 2 drops almond extract*

> *1 tablespoon sliced almonds*

Core the pears from the bottom, using a melon baller; leave the stem in place. Do not peel.

Bring the wine, water, peppercorns, cloves, and cinnamon stick to a boil in a non-reactive saucepan. Add the pears and more water, if necessary, to cover the pears.

Reduce the heat to a simmer. Cover the pan and cook 10 to 15 minutes, until the pears are barely tender when tested with a knife in the blossom end. Remove the pears from the heat, uncover, and allow them to cool in the poaching liquid. Refrigerate until ready to serve.

To make the almond cream, in a small bowl, whisk together the sour cream, brown sugar, and almond liqueur. Cover and refrigerate until ready to serve.

To serve, spoon 2 tablespoons of the almond cream in the center of each of 4 dessert plates, smoothing into a puddle with the back of a spoon. Place a pear upright in the center of each and sprinkle with the almonds. Serve with a knife and fork for eating.

Makes 4 servings.

JOSLIN CHOICES: 2 carbohydrate (fruit)

PER SERVING: 223 calories (5% calories from fat), 1 g total fat (0 saturated fat), 3 g protein,
35 g carbohydrates, 6 g dietary fiber, 2 mg cholesterol, 35 mg sodium, 335 mg potassium

Orange-Kissed Strawberries

*B*efore we tasted these, we didn't think one could better the taste of a luscious, fully ripe fresh strawberry. These orange-kissed berries are truly spectacular on their own or topped with a dollop of crème fraîche. Pile them into your prettiest stemmed dessert dish or goblet for the best effect.

> *4 cups fresh strawberries*
> *1 tablespoon sugar*
> *grated zest of 1 orange*
> *3 tablespoons fresh orange juice*
> *½ tablespoon orange-flavored liqueur*

Wash and stem the berries. Cut in half lengthwise and arrange in a single layer in a shallow dish.

Whisk together the sugar, orange zest, orange juice, and orange liqueur. Pour over the strawberries. Cover and let stand at room temperature for 20 minutes before serving in stemmed dessert dishes.

Makes 4 servings.

JOSLIN CHOICES: 1 carbohydrate (fruit)

PER SERVING: 64 calories (7% calories from fat), 1 g total fat (0 saturated fat), 1 g protein,
15 g carbohydrates, 4 g dietary fiber, 0 cholesterol, 2 mg sodium, 444 mg potassium

Banana Cake

*T*his moist cake is delicious with nondairy frozen whipped topping, a few slices of strawberries on top, or as is with a fragrant cup of coffee. Do use very ripe bananas when preparing any banana cake, as they are sweet and easy to mash. The aerosol baker's spray comes with flour, making it easy to coat your baking pan.

aerosol baker's spray with flour
3 bananas, mashed (about 1¼ cups)
⅓ cup canola oil
3 egg whites
¼ cup egg substitute
1 cup plain low-fat yogurt
2 cups unbleached all-purpose flour, sifted
3 tablespoons sugar
3 packets sugar substitute
2 teaspoons baking soda
2 teaspoons baking powder
1 teaspoon ground cinnamon
¼ teaspoon ground allspice
¼ teaspoon ground nutmeg
¼ cup finely chopped walnuts

Preheat the oven to 350°F. Lightly coat a 13 x 9-inch metal baking pan with aerosol baker's spray.

In a large bowl, beat together the bananas, oil, egg whites, egg substitute, and yogurt. Add the flour, sugar, sugar substitute, baking soda, baking powder, cinnamon, allspice, and nutmeg. Mix until combined. Fold in the nuts.

Pour into the prepared pan. Bake for about 25 to 30 minutes, until browned and the cake tests done. Cool and cut into 20 squares.

Makes 20 servings.

JOSLIN CHOICES: I carbohydrate (bread/starch), I fat

PER SERVING: 121 calories (37% calories from fat), 5 g total fat (1 g saturated fat), 3 g protein, 16 g carbohydrates, 1 g dietary fiber, 1 mg cholesterol, 172 mg sodium, 136 mg potassium

Lemon Cake

*T*his cake lends itself to all kinds of garnishes. Cut it in half and fill with nonfat sugarless frozen whipped topping and fresh or thawed frozen sliced berries for a festive dessert. Or serve it plain with hot tea for an afternoon treat.

aerosol baker's spray with flour (see page 212)
3 tablespoons reduced-fat margarine
¾ cup egg substitute
3 tablespoons sugar
5 packets sugar substitute
¼ cup very hot water
1 tablespoon fresh lemon juice
½ teaspoon vanilla extract
1 teaspoon grated lemon zest
1½ cups cake flour, sifted
2 teaspoons baking powder
6 large egg whites
pinch of salt

Preheat the oven to 325°F. Lightly coat a nonstick 10-inch springform pan with aerosol baker's spray.

Melt the margarine and set aside to cool. Beat the egg substitute until creamy and light. Continue to beat and add the sugar and sugar substitute slowly, until the mixture is pale and fluffy. Slowly add the water, lemon juice, cooled margarine, vanilla extract, and lemon zest. Combine the flour and baking powder. Sift over the batter and fold in gently, using as few strokes as possible.

Beat the egg whites with the salt until they hold stiff peaks. Gently fold the whites into the batter, trying not to deflate them. Place in the prepared pan. Bake for 40 to 45 minutes, until browned and the cake tests done. Cool in the pan on a rack. Remove the sides of the pan and cut into slices to serve.

Makes 12 servings.

JOSLIN CHOICES: 1 carbohydrate (bread/starch)
PER SERVING: 112 calories (22% calories from fat), 3 g total fat (0 saturated fat), 5 g protein,
  17 g carbohydrates, 0 dietary fiber, 0 cholesterol, 109 mg sodium, 96 mg potassium

Star Fruit Upside-Down Cake

Star fruit (carambola) makes a spectacular-looking dessert when baked in a brown sugar glaze with an orange-scented cake.

1 tablespoon reduced-fat margarine
1 tablespoon dark brown sugar
2 tablespoons fresh orange juice
3 large star fruit

CAKE
1¼ cups cake flour
¼ cup sugar
1 teaspoon baking powder
¼ teaspoon salt
2 large eggs, lightly beaten
2 tablespoons canola oil
1 teaspoon vanilla extract
½ cup fresh orange juice

Preheat the oven to 350°F.

Melt the margarine in a 9-inch round ovenproof skillet or round cake pan. Stir in the brown sugar until it dissolves. Stir in the orange juice. Slice each star fruit into 8 crosswise slices. Arrange the slices over the bottom of the pan, overlapping the slices as necessary to fit.

To make the cake, sift together the flour, sugar, baking powder, and salt in a medium mixing bowl. In a separate bowl, beat together the eggs, oil, vanilla extract, and orange juice. Pour over the dry ingredients and beat until smooth. Pour the batter over the star fruit and bake for 25 to 30 minutes, until a tester inserted in the center comes out clean.

Remove from the oven and run a knife around the edges of the cake to loosen it. Immediately invert onto a serving plate. Leave the baking dish on the cake for at least 5 minutes to allow the orange glaze to drain onto the cake. Remove the pan and scrape out any fruit or glaze that clings to the pan. Patch onto the top of the cake. Serve warm or at room temperature.

Makes 8 servings.

JOSLIN CHOICES: 2 carbohydrate (1 bread/starch, 1 fruit), 1 fat
PER SERVING: 191 calories (28% calories from fat), 6 g total fat (1 g saturated fat), 4 g
    protein, 31 g carbohydrates, 2 g dietary fiber, 53 mg cholesterol, 136 mg sodium, 177 mg
    potassium

Apple Strudel

The aroma of apples and cinnamon is synonymous with hearth and home. Here we make a festive dessert that's special enough for company yet easy to prepare for a family dinner. When pears are in season, use them and replace the orange juice and zest with lemon or, for a summer treat, use black plums. The variations are limitless. Add a few chopped nuts for crunch, currants macerated in sherry for a bit of sophistication, or use apple brandy instead of the orange juice.

butter-flavored cooking spray
3 Granny Smith apples, peeled, cored, and thinly sliced
1 tablespoon fresh orange juice
grated zest from ½ navel orange
sugar substitute equal to ¼ cup sugar or less, depending on your taste

1 teaspoon ground cinnamon
1 12-ounce sheet frozen puff pastry, thawed according to package directions
1 teaspoon sugar

Preheat the oven to 425°F. Line a baking sheet with parchment paper.

Lightly coat a nonstick skillet with cooking spray. Add the apples and sauté over medium heat for 2 minutes. Add the orange juice, zest, and sugar substitute.

Continue to sauté until the apples just begin to soften. Stir in ½ teaspoon cinnamon. Set aside.

Roll out the thawed pastry on a lightly floured board until it is ⅛ inch thick. Place the apples along one of the long sides. Roll up the pastry and apples to form a strudel roll. Place it on the prepared baking sheet, seam side down.

With a sharp knife, make horizontal slits every 2 inches. Combine the sugar with the remaining ½ teaspoon cinnamon and sprinkle over the top. Bake until deep golden and puffed, about 25 minutes. Let the strudel stand for 5 minutes before slicing. Serve warm.

Makes 8 servings.

JOSLIN CHOICES: 1 carbohydrate (fruit)
PER SERVING: 60 calories (31% calories from fat), 2 g total fat (1 g saturated fat), 1 g protein,
    11 g carbohydrates, 1 g dietary fiber, 0 cholesterol, 15 mg sodium, 68 mg potassium

Individual Peach Tarts

*F*ilo dough is a staple in our kitchens, purchased fresh at our local Greek market or frozen from the supermarket. With some fresh fruit, it makes a quick low-fat dessert with little effort. You may also make these tarts using apples, pears, nectarines, or plums.

4 18 x 14-inch filo dough sheets
butter-flavored cooking spray
4 firm ripe peaches, peeled and thinly sliced
grated zest of 1 lemon
½ teaspoon ground cinnamon

Preheat the oven to 375°F. If the filo dough is frozen, thaw it at room temperature following package directions. (Do not leave uncovered for more than a few minutes; it will dry out.)

Cut the filo dough into 4-inch squares. Working with 2 squares at a time (keep the remaining dough covered with a damp paper towel), place 2 squares on a work surface. Lightly coat each square with cooking spray and top each with another square. Lightly coat the top with cooking spray and continue adding layers of dough and lightly coating the tops with cooking spray until each square is stacked 6 layers deep. Transfer the stacks to a nonstick baking pan. Continue forming stacks until 8 are made.

Top each stack with half a peach, fanning out the slices. Sprinkle with lemon zest and cinnamon. Turn the corners up and over. (This allows the corners to brown nicely and gives the tarts a lovely shape.) Lightly spray each tart with cooking spray.

Bake until the filo is golden and the peaches are cooked through, about 15 minutes. Serve warm.

Makes 8 servings.

JOSLIN CHOICES: 1 carbohydrate (fruit)
PER SERVING: 65 calories (12% calories from fat), 1 g total fat (0 saturated fat), 1 g protein,
    13 g carbohydrates, 2 g dietary fiber, 0 cholesterol, 69 mg sodium, 111 mg potassium

Buttermilk Strawberry Cobbler

This is an easy dessert that can be baked and served still hot from the oven. The cobbler dough is dropped on top to form tender biscuits.

butter-flavored cooking spray

STRAWBERRY FILLING
6 cups fresh strawberries, hulled and cut into quarters
1 tablespoon sugar
finely grated zest of 1 lemon
1 tablespoon fresh lemon juice

BISCUIT TOPPING
1¾ cups unbleached all-purpose flour
1 tablespoon baking powder
1 teaspoon baking soda
1 tablespoon sugar
5 tablespoons reduced-fat margarine
1 cup fat-free buttermilk

Preheat the oven to 375°F. Lightly coat a 10-inch round or oval baking dish with cooking spray.

To make the filling, in a bowl, gently combine the strawberries, sugar, lemon zest, and lemon juice. Spoon the mixture into the prepared baking dish and bake for 10 minutes, until the juices begin to bubble around the edges.

In the meantime, make the topping. In a medium bowl, combine the flour, baking powder, baking soda, and ½ tablespoon sugar. Using a pastry blender or your fingers, work in the margarine until the mixture forms coarse crumbs. Stir in the buttermilk until the dry ingredients are just evenly moistened. Drop the dough by large spoonfuls onto the hot fruit, making 6 small rounds about ½ inch apart. Sprinkle the top of the dough with the remaining ½ tablespoon sugar.

Continue to bake until the dough is cooked through and the top is lightly browned, about 20 to 25 minutes. To serve, place a biscuit on each of 6 dessert bowls. Top each with some of the hot fruit and juice.

Makes 6 servings.

JOSLIN CHOICES: 3 carbohydrate (2 bread/starch, 1 fruit), 1 fat
PER SERVING: 273 calories (23% calories from fat), 7 g total fat (2 g saturated fat), 7 g
    protein, 47 g carbohydrates, 4 g dietary fiber, 1 mg cholesterol, 362 mg sodium, 608 mg
    potassium

Chocolate Mousse

*T*here are many recipes for low-fat mousses, but this one actually has the texture of the classic dessert. For extra flavor and kick, add 2 teaspoons of Kahlua or other coffee-flavored liqueur.

1 14-ounce container firm tofu, drained and pressed (see page 179)
¼ cup mocha-flavored sugar-free coffee mix
¼ cup plus 1 tablespoon unsweetened cocoa powder
1 to 1½ teaspoons ground cinnamon, to taste
1 12-ounce container frozen "free" nondairy whipped topping, thawed

Place the tofu in a food processor fitted with a metal blade; add the coffee mix, cocoa powder, and cinnamon. Blend until the mixture is smooth. Use a spatula to wipe down the sides of the work bowl.

Add the whipped topping and continue to process. Refrigerate until ready to serve.

Makes 9 servings.

JOSLIN CHOICES: 1½ carbohydrate (bread/starch), 1 fat
PER SERVING: 180 calories (36% calories from fat), 7 g total fat (5 g saturated fat), 5 g
    protein, 23 g carbohydrates, 0 dietary fiber, 1 mg cholesterol, 84 mg sodium, 193 mg
    potassium

Custard with Fresh Cherries

*I*n France this is called *clafouti aux cerises* and has been a staple for generations. When fresh cherries are in season, this is a refreshing light dessert. Try substituting fresh raspberries or any other berries, or even chopped pitted fruit, for a dessert that always pleases.

In addition to deep maroon Bing or Lambert cherries, other sweet varieties we use are golden Rainiers or the golden, red-blushed Royal Anns.

butter-flavored cooking spray
¼ cup unbleached all-purpose flour
sugar substitute equivalent to ¼ cup sugar
1 cup skim milk
1 cup evaporated skim milk
1 cup egg substitute
½ teaspoon ground cinnamon
⅛ teaspoon ground nutmeg
2 cups fresh sweet cherries, pitted

Preheat the oven to 350°F. Lightly coat a 10-inch pie pan or baking dish with cooking spray.

In a medium bowl, combine the flour and sugar substitute. Add both milks and the egg substitute. Beat until smooth. Stir in the cinnamon, nutmeg, and cherries.

Pour the mixture into the prepared dish and bake for 35 to 40 minutes, until the custard is brown and set.

Makes 8 servings.

JOSLIN CHOICES: 1 very-low-fat protein, 1 carbohydrate (fruit)
PER SERVING: 101 calories (14% calories from fat), 2 g total fat (0 saturated fat), 8 g protein, 15 g carbohydrates, 1 g dietary fiber, 2 mg cholesterol, 108 mg sodium, 343 mg potassium

Basic Sorbet Recipe

4 cups seeded fruit, melon, or berries
4 to 6 ice cubes
juice or zest of 1 lemon or lime, to taste, or fresh herbs such as mint or thyme
sugar substitute to taste (optional)

Place the fruit in a food processor fitted with a metal blade or in a blender, along with the lemon or lime juice or fresh herbs, and blend. Add artificial sweetener (if using). If desired, strain the mixture. Place in an ice cream maker and follow its directions until frozen. If freezing in ice cube trays, follow the directions below. Serve in dessert glasses.

Sorbet

*S*orbet is a refreshing way to end a meal. It can be made from any fruit or juice you have on hand, but don't stop there. You can also make it from brewed espresso or hot chocolate. Above is our master recipe. Add lemon or lime juice to sweet fruit, or for a different taste, add fresh mint or fresh thyme leaves. Just look at the Joslin Choices lists (starting on page 233) to find out how many carbohydrates you are using for the sorbet.

You can use an ice cream maker to make sorbet or use an ice cube tray, stirring the mixture every 20 minutes to break up crystals until the mixture freezes. The result will brighten your day.

Lemon Biscotti

A favorite dessert at our homes is a cup of freshly brewed espresso and a crisp Italian cookie, called biscotti. This version is tangy with fresh lemon and oh so good!

1¼ cups unbleached all-purpose flour
½ cup spoonable sugar substitute
1 teaspoon baking powder
3 tablespoons cold reduced-fat stick margarine, cut into bits
1 large egg or ¼ cup egg substitute
3 tablespoons grated lemon zest
3 tablespoons fresh lemon juice

Preheat the oven to 325°F. Line a baking sheet with parchment paper.

In a food processor, combine the flour, sugar substitute, and baking powder. Add the margarine and pulse until the mixture forms fine crumbs. Add the egg, lemon zest, and lemon juice. Pulse until the mixture forms a dough around the blade.

Turn the dough out onto a lightly floured work surface. Knead 2 or 3 times, adding more flour if needed (the dough should be sticky). Form the dough into a log about 2 inches in diameter. Transfer the log to the prepared baking sheet. Bake for 20 minutes.

Remove from the oven and let cool on the baking sheet on a rack for 15 minutes. Reduce the oven temperature to 275°F.

With a sharp knife, cut the log diagonally into ½-inch-thick slices. Then cut each slice in half. Arrange the half slices, standing upright, on the baking sheet and bake for another 10 minutes. Transfer the biscotti to wire racks to cool. Once cool, store in an airtight container until ready to serve.

Makes 36 biscotti, or 18 servings.

JOSLIN CHOICES (2 biscotti): I carbohydrate (bread/starch)
PER SERVING: 55 calories (19% calories from fat), I g total fat (0 saturated fat), I g protein,
   12 g carbohydrates, 0 dietary fiber, 0 cholesterol, 41 mg sodium, 33 mg potassium

Oatmeal-Raisin Cookies

These are chewy cookies—not too sweet, with a pleasing texture for young children. They are best eaten still warm from the oven.

   1 cup unbleached all-purpose flour
   ½ teaspoon baking soda
   ¼ teaspoon ground cinnamon
   ⅛ teaspoon salt
   ⅓ cup reduced-fat margarine, at room temperature
   ¼ cup spoonable brown sugar substitute
   3 tablespoons packed light brown sugar
   2 tablespoons granulated sugar
   1 large egg
   3 tablespoons skim milk

½ teaspoon pure vanilla extract
1½ cups rolled oats
½ cup dark raisins

Preheat the oven to 350°F. Line a large baking sheet with parchment paper.

On a piece of waxed paper, sift together the flour, baking soda, cinnamon, and salt. Set aside.

Using an electric mixer on medium speed, cream the margarine, brown sugar substitute, brown sugar, and granulated sugar until light and fluffy. Add the egg, milk, and vanilla. Beat well. Gradually add the flour mixture, ¼ cup at a time, beating after each addition.

By hand, stir in the oats and raisins. Drop by rounded teaspoonfuls onto the prepared baking sheet at least 2 inches apart. Bake until golden brown, about 10 to 12 minutes. Transfer the cookies to wire racks to cool.

Makes 36 cookies, or 18 servings.

JOSLIN CHOICES (2 cookies): 1 carbohydrate (bread/starch)
PER SERVING: 103 calories (26% calories from fat), 3 g total fat (1 g saturated fat), 2 g
     protein, 19 g carbohydrates, 1 g dietary fiber, 12 mg cholesterol, 92 mg sodium, 92 mg
     potassium

Spa Brownies

This recipe is adapted from the one used by Michael Stroot at the fabulous California Golden Door Spa and its sister spa, Rancho La Puerta, in nearby Mexico, a favorite after-holiday recuperation destination for us and our literary agent.

vegetable cooking spray
¾ cup unbleached all-purpose flour
½ cup unsweetened cocoa powder
1 teaspoon baking powder
½ teaspoon baking soda
⅓ cup mashed banana

6 tablespoons light brown sugar

6 tablespoons spoonable brown sugar substitute

½ cup unsweetened apple juice

1 teaspoon pure vanilla extract

½ teaspoon chocolate extract

4 large egg whites, at room temperature

½ teaspoon salt

¼ cup low-fat chocolate chips

Preheat the oven to 350°F. Lightly coat an 8-inch square baking pan with cooking spray.

In a medium bowl, sift together the flour, cocoa powder, baking powder, and baking soda. Set aside.

In a food processor or blender, combine the banana, brown sugar, brown sugar substitute, apple juice, vanilla extract, and chocolate extract. Process until smooth. Fold into the dry ingredients.

In a bowl, using an electric mixer on medium-high speed, beat the egg whites and salt until foamy. Increase the speed to high and beat until soft peaks form. Fold one-third of the egg whites into the banana-flour mixture to lighten it. Fold in the remaining egg whites.

Transfer the mixture to the prepared baking pan, smoothing the top with the back of a spoon. Bake for 30 to 35 minutes, until the brownie springs back when gently pressed in the center. Cool in the pan on a rack.

Place the chocolate chips in a 2-cup glass measuring cup. Microwave for about 30 seconds, until melted. Drizzle the chocolate over the brownies. Cut into 12 squares and serve.

Makes 12 servings.

JOSLIN CHOICES (1 brownie): 2 carbohydrate (bread/starch)

PER SERVING: 106 calories (9% calories from fat), 1 g total fat (1 g saturated fat), 3 g protein, 26 g carbohydrates, 2 g dietary fiber, 0 cholesterol, 193 mg sodium, 166 mg potassium

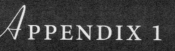

APPENDIX 1

Menus for 1,500 Calories

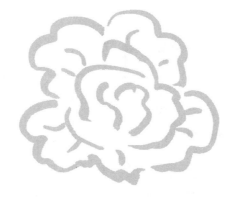

WEEK ONE	*Monday*	*Tuesday*	*Wednesday*
BREAKFAST 3 carbohydrate choices	1 serving Cheese and Herb Pancakes (page 114) 1 teaspoon soft margarine 1 cup sliced fresh strawberries	½ white grapefruit 1 Oatmeal Yogurt Muffin (page 116) 1 teaspoon soft margarine 8 fluid ounces skim milk	1 serving Country-Style French Toast (page 115) 2 teaspoons soft margarine ¾ cup fresh blueberries
LUNCH 3 carbohydrate choices	1 serving Grilled Portobello Mushroom Burger (page 95) 1 serving Hearts of Romaine with Basil-Yogurt Dressing (page 48) 8 fluid ounces skim milk 1 medium apple with peel	1 serving Golden Summer Frittata with Tomato Sauce (page 180) 1 serving Watermelon Salad (page 57)	1 serving Cold Yogurt and Garden Vegetable Soup (page 73) 1 serving Tomato and Mango Salad on Arugula and Curly Endive (page 55)
SNACK 1 carbohydrate choice	1 serving Baby Zucchini with Low-Fat Goat Cheese (page 34) 6 saltine crackers	¼ ounce dry-roasted salted almonds 1 serving Bananas Havana (page 208)	1 medium apple with peel 4 fluid ounces skim milk
DINNER 3 carbohydrate choices	1 serving Thai Noodles with Tofu and Peanuts (page 136) 1 serving Asian Vegetable Salad (page 68) 1 Oatmeal-Raisin Cookie (page 222)	1 serving Seasoned Bean Dip (page 29) 1 serving Baked Pita Chips (page 27) 1 serving Barley Risotto with Portobello Mushrooms (page 143) 1 serving Green Beans with Pistachios (page 192)	Pumpkin Ravioli with Mushroom Ragout (page 130) Mixed Citrus Salad (page 51) Belgian Endive with Herbed Ricotta (page 30)
SNACK 1 carbohydrate choice	1 ounce sliced low-fat cheddar cheese 6 unsalted saltine crackers	1 serving Mushrooms Stuffed with Garlic Mashed Potatoes (page 31) 1 ounce low-fat cheddar cheese	1 tablespoon unsalted chunky peanut butter 6 unsalted saltine crackers

Thursday	Friday	Saturday	Sunday
1 Raspberry Yogurt Muffin (page 117) 1 teaspoon soft margarine ¼ cup 2% fat cottage cheese 4 fluid ounces fresh orange juice	1 serving Wild Mushroom and Farmer's Cheese Omelet (page 107)	1 serving Curried Couscous with Walnuts (page 144) 8 fluid ounces skim milk	1 large egg, scrambled 2 slices whole wheat bread, toasted 1 teaspoon soft margarine ½ fresh white grapefruit
1 serving Mixed Mushroom Pizza (page 111) 1 cup tossed green salad 2 tablespoons Basic Oil and Vinegar Vinaigrette (page 69)	1 serving Stacked Cake Sandwich (page 102) 1 serving Herb-Roasted Tomato Soup (page 79)	1 serving Soupe au Pistou (page 83)	1 serving Bean and Pasta Soup (page 75) 1 serving Peach and Sweet Onion Salad (page 54)
1 serving Custard with Fresh Cherries (page 219)	1 serving Apple Strudel (page 215) 1 ounce low-fat cheddar cheese	1 cup cantaloupe cubes 4 ounces plain low-fat yogurt	3 graham crackers 1 tablespoon unsalted chunky peanut butter
1 serving Chickpeas and Tomato, Persian-Style (page 173) 1 serving Broccoli, Italian-Style (page 183) 1 serving Spinach Roulade (page 200)	1 serving Rigatoni with Lemon-Parsley Pesto (page 125) 1 serving Italian Roasted Beet Salad (page 57)	1 serving Zucchini Lasagna (page 205) 1 serving Italian Bread Salad (page 67)	1 serving Eggplant and Tomato Tart (page 188) 1 serving Poached Pears with Almond Cream (page 210)
1 ounce walnut halves ¾ cup fresh pineapple chunks	1 ounce unsalted bread sticks 1 tablespoon unsalted chunky peanut butter	1 serving Grilled Tofu Sandwiches (page 100)	1 serving Spicy Lentil Dip (page 28) 1 serving Baked Pita Chips (page 27)

WEEK TWO	*Monday*	*Tuesday*	*Wednesday*
BREAKFAST 3 carbohydrate choices	1 serving Refried Spicy Black Beans (page 169) 1 large egg, poached 1½ cups diced cantaloupe	1 cup cooked Quick Cream of Wheat cereal 2 teaspoons soft margarine 8 fluid ounces skim milk 1 medium orange	8 ounces cooked oat bran cereal 1 teaspoon soft margarine 8 fluid ounces skim milk 1 medium Bartlett pear
LUNCH 3 carbohydrate choices	1 serving Lentil Sandwiches with Spinach and Feta (page 105)	1 serving Eggplant and Tomato Pizza (page 110) 1 serving Apple and Jicama Salad (page 50)	1 serving Cuban Black Beans over Broiled Papaya (page 171) 1 cup tossed green salad 2 tablespoons Basic Oil and Vinegar Vinaigrette (page 69) 1 slice whole wheat bread 1 teaspoon soft margarine
SNACK 1 carbohydrate choice	½ ounce oil-roasted cashews 17 seedless grapes	4 ounces plain low-fat yogurt ½ serving Chocolate Popcorn (page 42)	2 unsalted rice cakes 2 tablespoons unsalted chunky peanut butter
DINNER 3 carbohydrate choices	1 serving Stuffed Pasta with Tomato Mushroom Sauce (page 139) 1 serving Spinach and Tempeh Salad with Wasabi Dressing (page 66)	1 serving Fettuccine with Garlic and Broccoli Rabe (page 120) 1 cup tossed green salad 1 tablespoon Dijon Mustard salad dressing (page 70)	1 serving Pasta Primavera with Sun-Dried Tomatoes (page 134) 1 Individual Peach Tart (page 216)
SNACK 1 carbohydrate choice	½ plain bagel (3½-inch diameter) 1 tablespoon unsalted chunky peanut butter	1 serving Lemon Cake (page 213) 2 tablespoons nondairy whipped topping 4 fluid ounces skim milk	¼ cup 1% fat cottage cheese 6 unsalted saltine crackers

Thursday	Friday	Saturday	Sunday
2 slices whole wheat bread, toasted 2 teaspoons soft margarine 2 teaspoons reduced-sugar jelly 1 large egg, poached 1 cup fresh raspberries	1 serving Couscous with Three Vegetables (page 145) ½ banana 1 hard-boiled egg 1 teaspoon soft margarine	1 homemade waffle (7-inch diameter) 1 teaspoon soft margarine 1 tablespoon reduced-calorie maple syrup ¼ cup 1% fat cottage cheese 1 cup sliced fresh strawberries	1 serving Country-Style French Toast (page 115) 2 teaspoons soft margarine 4 fluid ounces skim milk
1 serving Tortilla Soup (page 81) 1 serving Apricot and Orange Fool (page 207) 1 cup tossed green salad 1 tablespoon Basic Oil and Vinegar Vinaigrette (page 69)	1 serving Italian Pantry Soup with Basil Roasted Tomatoes (page 78) 1 serving Veggie Sandwich (page 101)	1 serving Vegetable Chili (page 84) 1 serving Belgian Endive and Watercress Salad (page 46)	1 serving Stuffed Pita Sandwiches (page 104) 1 medium apple with peel
¾ serving Mixed Berry Yogurt Smoothie (page 43)	¾ cup fresh tangerine (Mandarin orange) sections 4 ounces plain low-fat yogurt	1 Oatmeal-Raisin Cookie (page 222) 4 fluid ounces skim milk	3 graham crackers 2 tablespoons unsalted chunky peanut butter
1 serving Sweet-and-Sour Stuffed Cabbage (page 163) 1 serving Vegetable Tofu Kebobs (page 179)	1 serving Cold Rice Noodle Salad with Peanut Dressing (page 129) 1 serving Slow-Roasted Plum Tomatoes (page 202)	1 serving Polenta Lasagna (page 151) 1 cup tossed green salad 2 tablespoons Basic Vinegar and Oil Vinaigrette (page 69)	1 serving Refried Spicy Black Beans (page 169) 1 serving Braised Celery (page 184) 1 serving Fruited Gazpacho (page 72)
1 serving Banana Cake (page 212) 4 fluid ounces skim milk	1 medium apple with peel 1 ounce low-fat cheddar cheese	1 ounce pretzels 1 ounce low-fat processed American cheese	½ plain English muffin, toasted 1 ounce low-fat processed American cheese 2 slices raw tomato, ¼ inch thick 1 teaspoon olive oil

WEEK THREE	*Monday*	*Tuesday*	*Wednesday*
BREAKFAST 3 carbohydrate choices	1 cup cooked enriched farina cereal 2 teaspoons soft margarine 8 fluid ounces skim milk 4 fluid ounces low-calorie cranberry juice cocktail	1 cup cooked yellow grits 1 ounce low-sodium, low-fat cheddar cheese, diced 2 teaspoons soft margarine 8 fluid ounces skim milk	½ cup bran flakes cereal ½ medium banana 1 tablespoon whole blanched almonds 8 fluid ounces skim milk
LUNCH 3 carbohydrate choices	1 serving Sun-Dried Tomato and Lentil Soup (page 80) 1 serving Root and Vegetable Slaw with Lemon Dressing (page 62)	1 serving Artichoke and Feta Pizza (page 108) 1 cup tossed green salad 1 tablespoon Dijon Mustard salad dressing (page 70) 17 seedless grapes	1 serving Quesadillas (page 97) 2 ounces Guacamole (page 99) 1 cup tossed green salad 2 tablespoons Basic Oil and Vinegar Vinaigrette (page 69) ¾ cup fresh pineapple chunks
SNACK 1 carbohydrate choice	15 Teddy Grahams Vanilla Snack Cookies 8 ounces nonfat fruit yogurt with low-calorie sweetener	½ cup fat-free, no-sugar-added vanilla ice cream 2 tablespoons chopped walnuts	¼ cup 1% fat cottage cheese ½ plain bagel (3½-inch diameter)
DINNER 3 carbohydrate choices	1 serving Cherry Tomatoes Stuffed with Hummus (page 33) 1 serving Dried and Fresh Mushrooms with Linguine (page 127) 1 serving Baby Zucchini with Low-Fat Goat Cheese (page 34) 1 serving Southwestern Corn and Peach Salad (page 52)	1 serving Acorn Squash with Garlic Custard (page 196) 1 serving Spinach and Tempeh Salad with Wasabi Dressing (page 66) 4 ounces low-calorie pudding	1 serving Confetti Risotto (page 157) 1 serving Asparagus Flan (page 182)
SNACK 1 carbohydrate choice	1 slice whole wheat bread 2 teaspoons soft margarine 1 ounce low-fat processed American cheese	4 fluid ounces skim milk 5 vanilla wafers	1 slice whole wheat bread 2 tablespoons unsalted chunky peanut butter ½ ounce low-calorie grape jelly

Thursday	Friday	Saturday	Sunday
¾ cup corn flakes 8 fluid ounces skim milk ½ medium banana 1 tablespoon chopped walnuts	1 serving Kasha with Mushrooms, Peppers, and Bow-Ties (page 146) 1¼ cups whole strawberries	2 vegetarian sausage links 2 slices whole wheat toast 2 teaspoons soft margarine ½ fresh mango	1 serving Wild Mushroom and Farmer's Cheese Omelet (page 107)
1 serving Grilled Tofu Sandwiches (page 100) 1 serving Star Fruit Upside-Down Cake (page 214)	1 serving White Pizza (page 112) 1 serving Hearts of Romaine with Basil-Yogurt Dressing (page 48) ¾ cup fresh pineapple chunks	1 serving Tunisian Potato, Cauliflower, and Chickpea Salad (page 60) 8 fluid ounces skim milk	1 serving Spanish Vegetable and Rice Medley (page 160) 1 slice whole wheat bread 1 teaspoon soft margarine 1 medium apple
6 whole wheat crackers 1 ounce low-fat cheddar cheese	1 serving Chocolate Mousse (page 219)	45 Goldfish crackers ¼ cup 1% cottage cheese	6 whole wheat crackers 1 ounce low-fat cheddar cheese
1 serving Baba Ghanoush Bruschetta (page 22) 1 serving Zucchini Lasagna (page 205) 1 cup tossed green salad 1 tablespoon Basic Oil and Vinegar Vinaigrette (page 69)	1 serving Eggplant Terrine with Basil Tomato Sauce (page 38) 1 serving Niçoise Salad (page 64)	1 serving Lentils with Spinach (page 174) 1 serving Southwestern Tabbouleh (page 162) 1 cup tossed green salad 2 tablespoons Creamy Tofu Salad Dressing (page 70)	Slow-Roasted Vegetable Stew (page 91) Green Salad with Herbs and Warm Goat Cheese (page 47)
1 serving Red Potato Nibbles (page 32) 1 serving Grilled Portobello Mushrooms over Spinach (page 59)	½ plain bagel (3½-inch diameter) 2 tablespoons unsalted chunky peanut butter 1 tablespoon low-calorie jelly	4 ounces low-fat frozen vanilla yogurt	¾ ounce salted twisted pretzels 4 ounces nonfat fruit yogurt with low-calorie sweetener

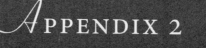
The Joslin Diabetes Food Lists for Meal Planning

The exchange categories that follow are different from those of a few years ago because of a new understanding about how food is metabolized. Today exchanges are grouped into Carbohydrates (bread/starch, fruit, milk, and vegetables—when consumed in sufficient quantities), Protein, and Fat. This new method allows for more individualized meal planning with your health-care team, taking into account your lifestyle, food likes and dislikes, medical conditions, and goals.

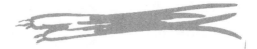

Carbohydrates List

A carbohydrate serving (approximately 15 grams) may include a food choice from the fruit, milk, and starch categories. Vegetables are also carbohydrates but contain fewer grams of carbohydrate (5 grams) per serving, so if you are using carbohydrate counting as your meal-planning option, be sure to note the difference.

Carbohydrate Choices

One choice provides:
CALORIES: 80
PROTEIN: 3 g
CARBOHYDRATE: 15 g
FAT: trace

Best choices:
Whole-grain breads and cereals,
dried beans, and peas.
(In general, one bread choice
equals 1 oz of bread.)

Breads

ITEM	PORTION
White, whole wheat, rye, etc.	1 slice (1 oz.)
Raisin, unfrosted	1 slice (1 oz)
Italian and French	1 slice (1 oz)
"Light"	
(1 slice equals 40 calories)	2 slices
Pita	
Pocket, 6-in. diameter	½ pocket
Mini size	1 pocket
Bagel	½ small (1 oz)
English muffin	½ small
Rolls	
Bulkie	½ small
Dinner, plain	1 small
Frankfurter	½ medium
Hamburger	½ medium
Bread crumbs	3 Tbsp.
Croutons	3 Tbsp.

Taco shells, small	2 (+ 1 Fat)
Tortilla, corn, 6-in. diameter	1
Tortilla, flour, 7-in. diameter	1 (+ 1 Fat)

Cereals

ITEM	PORTION
Cooked cereals	½ cup
Bran	
All-Bran with extra fiber*	1 cup
All-Bran*	⅓ cup
100% bran*	⅔ cup
40% bran flakes*	½ cup
Bran Chex*	½ cup
Fiber One*	⅔ cup
Multi-Bran Chex	⅓ cup
Cheerios*	1 cup
Common Sense Oat Bran	½ cup
Corn or Rice Chex	¾ cup
Cornflakes	¾ cup
Crispix	½ cup
Fortified Oak Flakes	½ cup
Frosted flakes	⅓ cup
Granola, low-fat	¼ cup
Grape-Nuts	3 Tbsp.
Grape-Nuts Flakes*	⅔ cup
Just Right (with nuggets)	¼ cup
Kix	1 cup
Life	½ cup
Nutri-Grain	½ cup
Product 19	½ cup
Puffed rice or wheat	1½ cups
Rice Krispies	⅔ cup

*High in fiber.

Shredded wheat biscuit*	1 cup
Spoon size	½ cup
Shredded Wheat 'n Bran*	½ cup
Special K	1 cup
Team	⅔ cup
Total	¾ cup
Wheat Chex*	½ cup
Wheaties*	⅔ cup

Starchy Vegetables

ITEM	PORTION
Corn	½ cup
Corn on the cob	1 small
Lima beans	½ cup
Mixed vegetables, with corn or peas	⅔ cup
Parsnips	½ cup
Peas, green, canned or frozen	⅔ cup
Plantain, cooked	⅓ cup
Potato, white	
Mashed	½ cup
Baked	½ medium or 1 small (3 oz)
Pumpkin	¾ cup
Sweet potato	
Mashed	⅓ cup
Baked	½ small or ½ cup (2 oz)
Winter squash, acorn or butternut	¾ cup

Pasta (cooked)

ITEM	PORTION
Macaroni, noodles, spaghetti	½ cup

High in fiber.

Legumes

ITEM	PORTION
Baked beans, canned, no pork (vegetarian-style)	⅓ cup
Beans, peas, lentils (cooked)	½ cup

Grains

ITEM	PORTION
Barley, cooked	⅓ cup
Bulgur, cooked	⅓ cup
Cornmeal	2½ Tbsp.
Cornstarch	2 Tbsp.
Couscous, cooked	⅓ cup
Flour	3 Tbsp.
Kasha, cooked	⅓ cup
Millet, dry	3 Tbsp.
Rice, cooked	⅓ cup
Wheat germ	¼ cup = 1 carb + 1 low-fat protein

Crackers

Best choices: Lower-sodium products, i.e., saltines with unsalted tops.

ITEM	PORTION
Ak-mak, regular and sesame	4 crackers
Animal crackers	8
Cheese Nips, reduced fat	22
Club, reduced fat	6
Finn Crisp	4
Gingersnaps	3
Graham crackers, 2½-in. squares	3
Granola bar, low-fat plain	1
Matzoh or matzoh with bran	1 (¾ oz)
Manischewitz whole wheat matzoh crackers	7

Melba toast rectangles	5
Melba toast rounds	10
Popcorn: popped, no fat added	3 cups
Orville Redenbacher Smart Pop!	4 cups
Pretzels*	7 regular or 12 mini
Mr. Phipps pretzel chips*	12
Rice cakes, popcorn cakes	2
Mini rice cakes	8
Ry-Krisp, triple crackers	3
Saltines*	6
Snack chips:*	
Baked potato or tortilla chips	15 small or 8 large (¾ oz)
SnackWell's, fat-free:	
Cheddar*	24
Cracked pepper*	8
Wheat*	6
Social Tea	4
Stella D'oro Almond Toast	2
Stella D'oro Egg Biscuit	2
Stoned Wheat Thins	3
Today's Choice water crackers	5
Town House, reduced fat	8
Triscuits, reduced fat	5
Uneeda	4
Wasa Lite or Golden Rye or Hearty Rye crispbread	2

Crackers for Occasional Use

(Equal to one starch **plus** one fat choice)

ITEM	PORTION
Arrowroot	4

*High in sodium.

Butter crackers*	
Rounds	7
Rectangular	6
Cheese Nips*	20
Cheez-It*	27
Club or Town House crackers*	6
Combos*	1 oz
Escort crackers*	5
Granola bar: plain, raisin, or peanut butter	1
Lorna Doone	3
Meal Mates*	5
Oyster crackers*	24
Peanut butter sandwich crackers*	3
Pepperidge Farm:	
Bordeaux cookies	3
Goldfish*	36
Popcorn, microwave light	4 cups
Ritz*	7
Sociables*	9
Stella D'oro Breakfast Treats	1
Stella D'oro Golden Bar	1
Stella D'oro Lady Stella Assortment	3
Stella D'oro Sesame Breadsticks	2
Sunshine HiHo*	6
Teddy Grahams	15
Tidbits*	21
Triscuits*	5
Vanilla wafers	6
Wasa Fiber Plus crispbread	4
Wasa Sesame or Breakfast crispbread	2
Waverly Wafers*	2
Wheat Thins, reduced fat*	13

High in sodium.

Fruit Choices

One choice provides: **Best choices:**

CALORIES: 60	Fresh whole fruit
PROTEIN: 0	**Be sure** to choose fresh, frozen, or canned fruit
CARBOHYDRATE: 15 g	packed in its own juice or water with no added
FAT: 0	sugar.

 Fruits

ITEM	PORTION
Apple, 2-in. diameter	1 small
Apple, dried	4 rings
Applesauce, unsweetened	½ cup
Apricots	
Fresh	4 medium
Canned	4 halves
Dried	7 halves
Banana, 9-in. length, peeled	½
Banana flakes or chips	3 Tbsp.
Blackberries	¾ cup
Blueberries	¾ cup
Boysenberries	1 cup
Canned fruit, unless otherwise stated	½ cup
Cantaloupe, 5-in. diameter	
Sectioned	⅓ melon
Cubed	1 cup
Casaba, 7-in. diameter	
Sectioned	⅙ melon
Cubed	1⅓ cups
Cherries	
Sweet fresh	12
Dried (no sugar added)	2 Tbsp.

Cranberries, dried (no sugar added)	2 Tbsp.
Currants	2 Tbsp.
Dates	3
Figs	
Fresh	2 small
Dried	1 small
Granadillas (passionfruit)	4
Grapefruit, 4-in. diameter	½
Grapes	15 small
Guavas	1½ small
Honeydew melon, 6½-in. diameter	
Sectioned	⅛ melon
Cubed	1 cup
Kiwifruit (3 oz)	1 large
Kumquats	5 medium
Loquats, fresh	12
Lychees, fresh or dried	10
Mango	½ small
Sliced	½ cup
Nectarine, 2½-in. diameter	1 small
Orange, 3-in. diameter	1 small
Papaya, 3½-in. diameter	
Sectioned	½
Cubed	1 cup
Peach, 2½-in. diameter	1 small
Pear	1 small
Persimmon	
Native	2
Japanese, 2½-in. diameter	½
Pineapple	
Fresh, diced	¾ cup
Canned, packed in juice	⅓ cup
Plaintain, cooked	⅓ cup
Plums, 2-in. diameter	2 small
Pomegranate, 3½-in. diameter	½

Prunes, dried, medium	3
Raisins	2 Tbsp.
Raspberries	1 cup
Rhubarb, fresh, diced	3 cups
Strawberries, whole	1⅓ cups
Tangerines, 2½-in. diameter	2 small
Watermelon, diced	1¼ cups

Fruit Juice

Be sure to monitor your blood glucose. Fruit juice may elevate blood glucose rapidly, especially when consumed on an empty stomach or with a small amount of food such as a snack. Limit your intake of juice to no more than one meal each day or to times when you are engaging in vigorous activity or treating a low blood sugar.

ITEM	PORTION
Apple juice, unsweetened	4 oz
Cranapple, unsweetened	3 oz
Cranberry, low-calorie	9 oz
Cranberry, unsweetened	4 oz
Grape juice, unsweetened	3 oz
Grapefruit juice, unsweetened	5 oz
Lemon juice	8 oz
Orange juice, unsweetened	4 oz
Pineapple juice, unsweetened	4 oz
Prune juice, unsweetened	3 oz
Twister Light (with aspartame)	15 oz
Twister, regular	4 oz

Vegetable Choices

One choice provides:
CALORIES: 25
PROTEIN: 2 g

Best choices:
Fresh raw vegetables: dark green, leafy, or orange.
Be sure to choose at least 2 vegetables each day.

CARBOHYDRATE: 5 g

FAT: 0

We encourage steaming with a minimum amount of water. The portion listed is for a **cooked** serving unless noted otherwise.

Vegetables

ITEM	PORTION
Artichoke	½
Asparagus	1 cup
Bamboo shoots	1 cup
Bean sprouts	½ cup
Beet greens	½ cup
Beets	½ cup
Broccoli	½ cup
Brussels sprouts	½ cup
Cabbage	1 cup
Carrots	½ cup
Cauliflower	1 cup
Celery	1 cup
Collard greens	1 cup
Eggplant	½ cup
Fennel leaf	1 cup
Green beans	1 cup
Green pepper	1 cup
Kale	½ cup
Kohlrabi	½ cup
Leeks	½ cup
Mushrooms, fresh	1 cup
Mustard greens	1 cup
Okra	½ cup
Onion	½ cup
Radishes	1 cup
Red pepper	1 cup

Rutabagas	½ cup
Sauerkraut*	½ cup
Snow peas (Chinese pea pods)	½ cup
Spinach	½ cup
Squash	
Spaghetti	½ cup
Summer	1 cup
Zucchini	1 cup
Swiss chard	1 cup
Tomato (ripe)	1 medium
Tomato, canned*	½ cup
Tomato juice or V8 juice	½ cup
Tomato paste*	1½ Tbsp.
Tomato sauce, canned	⅓ cup
Spaghetti sauce, jar	¼ cup
Turnip greens	1 cup
Turnips	½ cup
Vegetables, mixed	½ cup
Water chestnuts	6 whole or ¼ cup
Wax beans	½ cup

Because of their low carbohydrate and calorie content, the following **raw** vegetables may be used liberally:

Alfalfa sprouts	Lettuce, all types
Celery	Mushrooms
Chicory	Parsley
Chinese cabbage	Pickles (unsweetened)*
Cucumber	Pimiento
Endive	Spinach
Escarole	Watercress

*These vegetables are high in sodium (salt). Low-sodium vegetables, juices, and sauces should be purchased if you are following a sodium-restricted diet. Fresh and frozen vegetables are lower in sodium than canned vegetables, unless the canned product states "low sodium."

Milk Choices

Best choices: Nonfat or low-fat.

Be sure to take calcium supplements if you use less than 2 cups per day (adults) or 3–4 cups per day (children).

Nonfat Selections

One choice provides:
CALORIES: 90
PROTEIN: 8 g
CARBOHYDRATE: 12 g
FAT: 0

ITEM	PORTION
Nonfat milk (skim)	1 cup
Nonfat buttermilk	1 cup
½% milk	1 cup
Nonfat plain yogurt	¾ cup
Nonfat yogurt made with Aspartame, i.e., Yoplait Light, Weight Watchers Ultimate 90, Dannon Light	6–8 oz
Lactaid milk (skim)	1 cup
Powdered, nonfat milk, dry	⅓ cup
Canned, evaporated skim milk	½ cup
Sugar-free hot cocoa mix plus 6 oz of water*	1 cup

Most cocoa mixes do not provide the same amount of calcium as one cup of milk. Mixes that do provide the same amount should indicate on the label that the product contains 30% Daily Value for calcium. An example of a product that meets these calcium requirements is Alba sugar-free hot cocoa mix.

Low-Fat Selections

One choice provides:

CALORIES: 105
PROTEIN: 8 g
CARBOHYDRATE: 12 g
FAT: 3 g

ITEM	PORTION
1% milk	1 cup
1% buttermilk	1 cup
Yogurt, plain, unflavored	¾ cup
Lactaid milk (1%)	1 cup

Medium- and High-Fat Selections

One choice provides:

CALORIES: 120–150
PROTEIN: 8 g
CARBOHYDRATE: 12 g
FAT: 5–8 g

The following milk items should be used sparingly due to their high saturated fat and cholesterol content.

ITEM	PORTION
2% milk	1 cup
Whole milk	1 cup

Other Carbohydrates

Breakfast Items

ITEM	PORTION	FOOD GROUP	GRAMS CARB	CAL
Nutri-Grain bar	1	2 carbs + 1 fat	27 g	205
Muffin, bran or corn	small (2 oz)	1 carb + 1 fat	22 g	125

Muffin, from mix	¹⁄₁₂ of pkg.	1 carb + 1 fat	17 g	125
Weight Watchers blueberry muffin	1	2 carbs + 1 fat	33 g	205
Croissant	1 (2 oz)	2 carbs + 2 fat	25 g	250
Doughnut, cake-type	1 small (1 oz)	1 carb + 1 fat	12 g	125
Doughnut, frosted	1 (2 oz)	2 carbs + 2 fat	30 g	250
Sweet roll/danish	1 (2 oz)	2 carbs + 2 fat	28 g	250
Biscuit	1 (1 oz)	1 carb + 1 fat	13 g	125
Corn bread, from mix	1 (2 oz)	2 carbs + 1 fat	30 g	205
Pancake	2 (4-in. diam.)	1 carb	13 g	125
Waffle				
Homemade	4-in. diam.	1 carb + 0–1 fat	13 g	125
Frozen	4-in. diam.	1 carb + 1 fat	15 g	125
Granola				
Regular	¼ cup	1 carb + 1 fat	20 g	125
Low-fat	¼ cup	1 carb	16 g	80

Desserts

ITEM	PORTION	FOOD GROUP	GRAMS CARB	CAL
Angel food cake	¹⁄₁₂ of cake	2 carbs	30 g	160
Brownie, unfrosted	2-in. square	2 carbs + 1 fat	25 g	205
Cake, frosted	2 oz	3 carbs + 1 fat	40 g	285
Cookies:				
Fig Newtons, fat-free or regular	2	1 carb	22 g	80
SnackWell's fat-free:				
Creme-filled	2	1 carb	21 g	80
Chocolate truffle	1	1 carb	13 g	80
Devil's food or fudge	1	1 carb	13 g	80
Brownie	1	2 carbs	26 g	160
SnackWell's reduced-fat chocolate chip	15	1 carb	15 g	80
Cake, unfrosted	2 oz	2 carbs + 1 fat	35 g	205
Cupcake, frosted	1	2 carbs + 1 fat	28 g	205

Frozen dessert bars:				
Creamsicle, regular	1 bar	1 carb + 1 fat	19 g	125
Dole Fruit'n Cream, Bar	1 bar	1 carb	17 g	80
Dole Fruit'n Juice Bar, regular	1 bar	1 carb	16 g	80
Eskimo Pie Pudding Bar	1 bar	1 carb	15 g	80
Häagen-Dazs fat-free Sorbet 'n' Yogurt	1 bar	1 carb	20 g	80
Fudgsicle fudge bar, no sugar added	2 bars	1 carb	16 g	80
Push-up	1 bar	1 carb	20 g	80
Welch's Fruit Juice Bar:				
Regular	1 bar	1 carb	11 g	80
No sugar added	2 bars	1 carb	12 g	80
Weight Watchers:				
Chocolate mousse bar	2 bars	1 carb	18 g	80
Orange Vanilla Treat	2 bars	1 carb	17 g	80
Ice cream sandwich	1	2 carbs + 1 fat	30 g	205
Frozen yogurt (Edy's or Breyers):				
Low-fat	½ cup	1 carb + 1 fat	17 g	125
Fat-free	½ cup	1 carb	22 g	80
Fat-free, no sugar added	½ cup	1 carb	18 g	80
Ice cream (Edy's or Breyers):				
Regular	½ cup	1 carb + 2 fat	17 g	170
Low-fat or fat-free	½ cup	1 carb	22 g	80
No sugar added	½ cup	1 carb + 1 fat	15 g	125
Fat-free, no sugar added	½ cup	1 carb	19 g	80

Pudding:				
Sugar-free	½ cup	1 carb	14 g	80
Regular	½ cup	2 carbs	29 g	160
Sherbet, sorbet	½ cup	2 carbs	27 g	160

Miscellaneous

ITEM	PORTION	FOOD GROUP	GRAMS CARB	CAL
Jam/jelly, honey, regular	1 Tbsp	1 carb	13 g	80
Spaghetti sauce	½ cup	1 carb + 0 –1 fat	10 g	125
Sugar	1 Tbsp	1 carb	12 g	46
Syrup:				
Light	2 Tbsp	1 carb	13 g	80
Regular	2 Tbsp	2 carbs	27 g	160
Yogurt, fruited, regular	1 cup	3 carbs	45 g	240

"Free" Foods List

The following foods contain very few calories and may be used freely in your meal plan. Items marked with an asterisk (*) are high in sodium; you should check with your doctor or dietitian before using these products.

General:

Bouillon, broth, or consommé*
Chewing gum, sugar-free
Cocoa powder
Coffee, tea
Cranberries (unsweetened)
Extracts
Gelatin mixes, sugar-free
Herbs, seasonings, spices
Hot pepper sauce, taco sauce*

High in sodium.

Lemon/lime juice

Lemon/lime/orange rind

Noncaloric diet soft drinks, unsweetened seltzer waters

Pickles (unsweetened)*

Postum (limit to 3 cups daily)

Soy sauce, steak sauce*

Unprocessed bran (1 Tbsp.)

Vinegar

Many fat-free choices contain one or more types of sugar. The amount of sweetener is small; however, the portion used should be no more than the amount listed on this page or no more than *20 calories per serving,* approximately three times per day. Always read the labels carefully, and consult your physician or dietitian if you plan to use these items regularly.

Protein List

Best choices: Very-low-fat or low-fat selections.

Be sure to trim off visible fat. Bake, broil, or steam selections with no added fat. Weigh your portion after cooking.

We recommend that portions be the accompaniment rather than the main course.

Very-Low-Fat Selections

One choice provides:

CALORIES: 35–45

PROTEIN: 7 g

CARBOHYDRATE: 0

FAT: 0–2 g

ITEM	PORTION
Beef:	
Healthy Choice 96% fat-free ground beef	1 oz
Cheese products, fat-free:*	
Kraft Free, Alpine Lace slices	1 slice
Healthy Choice or Kraft shredded	3 Tbsp.

High in sodium.

Cottage cheese, fat-free or 1%*	¼ cup
Ricotta, 100% fat-free*	1 oz
Dried beans, cooked	½ cup = 1 protein + 1 carb
Egg substitute, plain (less than 40 calories per serving)	¼ cup
Egg whites	2
Fish and seafood: fresh or frozen cod, flounder, haddock, halibut, trout, tuna (in water); clams, crab, lobster, scallops, shrimp, imitation crabmeat	1 oz
Game, venison, buffalo, ostrich	1 oz
Ground turkey, 93–99% fat-free only	1 oz
Hot dogs, 97% fat-free*	1 oz
Luncheon meats:* 95% fat-free pastrami, ham, turkey ham, turkey bologna	1 oz
Poultry: chicken, turkey, or Cornish hen—white meat only and skinless	1 oz
Turkey sausage, 97% fat-free*	1 oz

Low-Fat Selections

One choice provides:

CALORIES: 55
PROTEIN: 7 g
CARBOHYDRATE: 0
FAT: 3 g

ITEM	PORTION
Beef:	
ground beef, 90% fat-free	1 oz
USDA Select or Choice grades of flank, round, sirloin, T-bone, tenderloin cuts	1 oz

High in sodium.

Cheeses:*

Cottage cheese, 4.5% fat	¼ cup
Kraft Light, slices	1 oz
Mozzarella, light	1 oz

Fish:

herring, uncreamed or smoked*	1 oz
Oysters, salmon, sardines (in tomato or mustard sauce*)	1 oz
Ground turkey or chicken, lean only	1 oz
Hot dogs, 90% fat-free*	1
Luncheon meats, 90% fat-free*	1 oz
Pork: lean only, center loin, fresh ham, loin chop, tenderloin	1 oz

Poultry:

Chicken or turkey, dark meat, no skin, or white meat with skin	1 oz
Tofu	3 oz
Turkey sausage, 90% fat-free*	1 oz
Veal: lean, trimmed only, loin chop, round	1 oz

Medium-Fat Selections

One choice provides:

CALORIES: 75

PROTEIN: 7 g

CARBOHYDRATE: 0

FAT: 5 g

ITEM	PORTION
Beef: chipped, chuck, flank steak; hamburger (90% fat-free), rib eye, rump, sirloin, tenderloin top and bottom round	1 oz

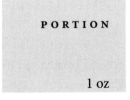

High in sodium.

Cheese:*	
part-skim mozzarella, part-skim Ricotta, farmer, Neufchâtel, Velveeta light, Jarlsberg Lite, Dorman's Slim Jack reduced-fat Monterey, Cracker Barrel light, Cabot light, Vitalait, Kraft Light	1 oz
Parmesan,* Romano	3 Tbsp.
Egg†	1
Egg substitute with 60–80 calories per ¼ cup	¼ cup
Lamb, except for breast	1 oz
Luncheon meat, "light" (turkey bologna, turkey pastrami)*	1 oz
Peanut butter	1 Tbsp. = 1 protein + 1 fat
Pork, except for deviled ham, ground pork, and spare ribs	1 oz
Turkey bacon	2 slices
Turkey franks, "light"	1 = 1½ protein
Veal, except for breast	1 oz

High-Fat Selections

One choice provides:
CALORIES: 100
PROTEIN: 7 g
CARBOHYDRATE: 0
FAT: 8 g

Be sure to use the meat choices listed below sparingly because of their high saturated fat and cholesterol content.

ITEM	PORTION
Beef: brisket, club and rib steak, corned beef,* regular hamburger with 20% fat, rib roast, short ribs	1 oz

*High in sodium.

†Eggs are high in cholesterol. Limit consumption to 3 or 4 per week.

Cheese, regular: blue,* brie, cheddar, Colby, feta,* Monterey Jack, Muenster, provolone, Swiss, pasteurized process*	1 oz
Fish, fried	1 oz
Hot dog, regular, beef or pork	1 oz = 1 protein + 1 fat
Lamb: breast	1 oz
Luncheon meats, regular:* bologna, bratwurst, braunschweiger, knockwurst, liverwurst, pastrami, Polish sausage, salami	1 oz
Organ meats: liver, heart, kidney	1 oz
Pork: deviled ham,* ground pork, spare ribs, sausage* (patty or link)	1 oz
Poultry: capon, duck, goose	1 oz
Veal: breast	1 oz

Fat List

One choice provides:

CALORIES: 45
PROTEIN: 0
CARBOHYDRATE: 0
FAT: 5 g

Best choices:

Monounsaturated fats. However, limit total amount of all types of fat.
Be sure when using a low-calorie version of fat choices to use amounts equal to 45 calories for one serving.

Monounsaturated Fats

ITEM	PORTION
Avocado, 4-in. diameter	⅛
Oils: canola, olive, peanut	1 tsp.
Olives:*	
Black	9 large
Green	10 large

High in sodium.

Nondairy creamer:

Liquid	2 Tbsp.
Reduced-fat liquid	5 Tbsp.

Nuts (unsalted):

almonds	6
Brazil	2
cashews	6
filberts (hazelnuts)	5
macadamia	3
mixed	6
peanuts, Spanish	20
peanuts, Virginia	10
pecans	4 halves
pignola (pine nuts)	1 Tbsp.
pistachio	12
Sesame seeds	1 Tbsp.
Tahini	2 tsp.

Polyunsaturated Fats

ITEM	PORTION
Margarine: stick, tub, or squeeze	1 tsp.
Reduced-fat	1 Tbsp.
Mayonnaise	1 tsp.
Reduced-fat	1 Tbsp.
Nuts: walnuts (unsalted)	4 halves
Oils: corn, cottonseed, safflower, soy, sunflower	1 tsp.
Salad dressings, regular:	
French,* 1,000 Island	1 Tbsp.
Italian*	2 tsp.
Creamy types	2 tsp.
Salad dressings, reduced-calorie:	
Italian*	2 Tbsp.
Ranch*	1 Tbsp.

*High in sodium.

Red wine vinegar & oil	2 Tbsp.
Seeds:* pumpkin, sunflower (unsalted)	1 Tbsp.

Saturated Fats

ITEM	PORTION
Bacon, cooked*	1 strip
Butter:	
Stick	1 tsp.
Whipped	2 tsp.
Reduced-fat	1 Tbsp.
Chitterlings	2 Tbsp. (½ oz)
Coconut, shredded	2 Tbsp.
Coffee whitener, liquid	2 Tbsp.
Coffee whitener, powder	4 Tbsp.
Cream:	
Half & half	2 Tbsp.
Heavy	1 Tbsp.
Light	1½ Tbsp.
Whipped	1 Tbsp.
Whipped, pressurized	⅓ cup
Cream cheese:	
Regular	1 Tbsp.
Reduced-fat	2 Tbsp.
Oils: coconut or palm	1 tsp.
Salt pork*	¼ oz
Shortening or lard	1 tsp.
Sour cream:	
Regular	2 Tbsp.
Reduced-fat	3 Tbsp.

*High in sodium.

One choice = a free exchange

ITEM	PORTION
Catsup*	1 Tbsp.
Cream cheese:	
Philadelphia Free	1 Tbsp.
Gravy:*	
Pepperidge Farm 98% fat-free gravy	3 Tbsp.
Heinz HomeStyle fat-free gravy	¼ cup
Hard candy or mints, sugar-free	3 or less
Jams:	
Smucker's Light Preserves	1 Tbsp.
Smucker's Simply 100% Fruit	1 tsp.
Polaner All Fruit	1 tsp.
Knott's Berry Farm light preserves	1 Tbsp.
Mayonnaise:	
Cain's Fat-Free Mayonnaise	1 Tbsp.
Kraft Fat-Free Mayonnaise	2 Tbsp.
Kraft Miracle Whip Free	1 Tbsp.
Margarine:	
Fleischmann's fat-free squeeze bottle	¼ cup
Promise Ultra spread	2 tsp.
Promise Ultra, fat-free spread	¼ cup
Butter Buds	1 Tbsp.
Molly McButter	1 Tbsp.
Nonstick pan sprays	5-second spray
"I Can't Believe It's Not Butter" pump spray	5 sprays
Mustard*	1 Tbsp.
Frozen dessert bars, no sugar added:	
Fudgsicle	1 bar
Welch's Fruit Juice Bar	1 bar

*High in sodium.

Salad dressings:

Good Seasons Fat-Free, all flavors	2 Tbsp.
Kraft Free:	
Italian	2 Tbsp.
Ranch, Blue cheese	1 Tbsp.
1,000 Island, Catalina	1 Tbsp.
Seven Seas Free:	
Italian or Red Wine Vinegar	2 Tbsp.
Wish-Bone Fat Free:	
Caesar, Creamy Roasted Garlic, Chunky Blue Cheese, French, 1,000 Island, Honey Dijon	1 Tbsp.
Wish-Bone Lite:	
Italian or 1,000 Island	2 Tbsp.
Hidden Valley:	
Blue Cheese	2 Tbsp.
Italian	2 Tbsp.
Caesar, Creamy Parmesan, Ranch, Honey Dijon	1 Tbsp.
Sour cream, fat-free	1 Tbsp.
Syrup:	
Cary's Sugar Free	2 Tbsp.
Fifty 50, reduced-calorie	1 Tbsp.

Combination Foods List

Many foods are made up of several food groups. These mixed foods can be incorporated into your meal plan by substituting them for choices from more than one food group.

Canned Soup *

ITEM	PORTION	FOOD GROUP	GRAMS CARB	CAL
Rice or noodle with broth, prepared with water	8 oz	1 carb	9 g	80
Chunky styles, ready to serve	8 oz	1 carb, 1 protein	12 g	135
Cream soup: made with water	8 oz	1 carb, 1 fat	9 g	125
Made with 1% low-fat milk	8 oz	1 carb, 1 fat	15 g	125
Clam chowder, New England style prepared with 1% low-fat milk	8 oz	1 carb, 1 fat	20 g	125
Lentil with ham, Ready to serve	8 oz	1 carb, 1 protein, 1 vegetable	20 g	160
Minestrone, ready to serve	8 oz	1 carb	16 g	80
Split pea with ham, ready to serve	8 oz	2 carb, 1 protein	28 g	215
Tomato, made with water	8 oz	1 carb	17 g	80
Vegetable made with water	8 oz	1 vegetable	8 g	25

*High in sodium unless specially prepared without salt. Brands to look for that have less fat and sodium are: Campbell's Healthy Request, Fantastic Foods (dried), Healthy Choice, Progresso Healthy Classics

Prepared Foods *

ITEM	PORTION	FOOD GROUP	GRAMS CARB	CAL
Beef stew, homemade	1 cup	2 protein, 1 carb	15 g	190
Chicken pot pie, frozen	7 oz	2½ carb, 1 protein, 1 vegetable, 4 fat	40 g	460
Chili with meat and beans, homemade	1 cup	2 protein, 1 carb	22 g	190
Lasagna, homemade	2½ x 2½ x 1¾ in.	2 carbs, 3 protein, 1 vegetable, 2 fat	35 g	215
Macaroni & cheese, made from package	1 cup	3 carb, 1 protein, 2 fat	45 g	385
Pizza, cheese*	⅛ of 14-in. diameter	1 carb, 1 protein, 1 vegetable, 1 fat	18 g	205
Ravioli, canned	1 cup (7 oz)	2 carb, 1 protein, 1 fat	30 g	260
Spaghetti with meat, canned*	1 cup	1 carb, 2 vegetable, 1 protein, 1 fat	26 g	230
Spaghetti with meatballs, homemade*	1 cup	2 carb, 2 protein	40 g	270
Taco, beef	1	2 protein, 1 carb, 1 fat	15 g	235

High in sodium unless specially prepared without salt.

Food Lists for Vegetarian Meal Planning

Carbohydrate Foods

Starch: Grains / Breads / Starchy Vegetables

SERVING = 1 carb *(15 g carb, 3 g protein)*

Corn/flour tortilla, 6 in.
Pita bread, ½ of 2 oz loaf
Miso, 3 Tbsp.

Cooked grains:

Barley, ⅓ cup	Oat bran, ¼ cup
Brown rice, ⅓ cup	Quinoa, ⅓ cup
Buckwheat, ½ cup	Wheat berries, ⅔ cup
Bulgur, ½ cup	Wild rice, ½ cup
Couscous, ⅓ cup	

Milk

SERVING = 1 carb and ½ to 2 fats *(15 g carb, 8 g protein, 2–10 g fat)*

Acidophilus milk, 1 cup	Kefir, 1 cup
Buttermilk, 1 cup	Rice milk, ½ cup
Goat milk, 1 cup	Soy milk, 1 cup

Vegetables

FREE for 1–2 servings; 5 g carb *(15 g carb for 3 servings)*

Bamboo shoots, ½ cup
Celeriac, raw, ½ cup
Endive, 1 medium head
Greens, ½ cup

Jicama, raw, ½ cup
Seaweed, 1 oz.
Sprouts, ½ cup

Meat Substitutes / Protein Foods

SERVING =1 protein *(0 g carb, 7 g protein, 0–5 fat)*

Egg substitute, ¼ cup
Soy cheese, 1 oz
Tofu, firm, ½ cup (4 oz)

Vegetarian breakfast links, 1 link (1 oz)*
Vegetarian breakfast patties, 1 patty (1.3 oz)*
Vegetarian hotdog, 1 (1.5 oz)*

Beans (cooked): SERVING = 1 carb + 1 lean protein *(15 g carb, 7 g protein)*

Black beans, ½ cup
Black-eyed peas, ½ cup
Chickpeas, garbanzo beans, ⅓ cup
Lentils, ½ cup

Lima beans, ½ cup
Navy, kidney, pinto beans, ⅓ cup
Refried beans, ½ cup
Split peas, ⅓ cup

Nuts/Seeds: SERVING = 1 protein + 2–3 fats *(0 carb, 7 g protein, 10–15 g fat)*

Almonds, pecans, peanuts, ¼ cup
Pine nuts, pignolias, 2 Tbsp
Pistachios, ¼ cup (1 oz)

Pumpkin or squash seeds, ¼ cup
Sesame or sunflower seeds, ¼ cup
Walnuts, 16–20 halves

Fat Foods

SERVING = 1 fat *(0 carb, 5 g fat)*

Almond butter: 1 Tbsp = 2 fat
Cashew butter: 1 Tbsp = 2 fat
Flax seed oil: 1 tsp = 1 fat

Peanut oil: 1 tsp = 1 fat
Sesame butter, tahini: 1 Tbsp = 2 fat

*Some vegetarian meat substitutes may also contain carbohydrate.

Combination Foods*

ITEM	PORTION	FOOD GROUP
Bean and cheese tostada	1 tostada (5 oz)	2 carbs, 1 protein, 3 fat
Falafel	3 patties (3 oz) 2 in. diam.	1 carb, 1 protein, 4 fat
Hummus	½ cup	1 carb, 1 protein, 2 fat
Tempeh	½ cup	1 carb, 2 protein
Textured vegetable protein	¾ oz	½ carb, 1 protein
Tofu-based ice cream	½ cup	1 carb, 2 fat
Vegetarian chili	⅔ cup	1 carb, 3 protein
Vegetarian "garden" burger	1 patty (2.5 oz)	1 carb, 1 protein
Vegetarian soy burger	1 patty (2.5 oz)	½ carb, 2 protein
Wheat germ, toasted	½ cup	1 carb, 1 protein, 2 fat

Helpful Hints:

1 carbohydrate choice = 15 grams carbohydrate

1 protein choice = 7 grams protein

1 fat choice = 5 grams fat

For more specific carbohydrate values of foods, read the food label or look up values in a carbohydrate counting book.

*Depending on the brand or preparation method, these foods may have additional fat.

$\mathcal{A}$PPENDIX 3

Joslin Diabetes Center and Its Satellites and Affiliates

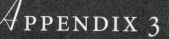

CONNECTICUT

Joslin Diabetes Center
Affiliate at New Britain General Hospital
> 100 Grand Street
> New Britain, CT 06050
> (888) 4-JOSLIN
> (860) 224-5672

Joslin Diabetes Center
Affiliate at Charlotte Hungerford Hospital
> Hungerford Building
> 540 Litchfield Street
> Torrington, CT 06790
> (860) 489-0661

Joslin Diabetes Center
Affiliate at Lawrence and Memorial Hospital
> 50 Faire Harbor Place
> Suite 2E
> New London, CT 06320
> (877) JOSLIN-1
> (860) 444-4737

FLORIDA

Joslin Diabetes Center
Affiliate at Morton Plant Mease Health Care
455 Pinellas Street
Clearwater, FL 34616
(satellite locations in Dunedin and Countryside)
(727) 461-8300

INDIANA

Floyd Memorial Hospital & Health Services
1850 State Street
New Albany, IN 47150
(812) 949-5700
(888) 77-FMHHS

MARYLAND

Joslin Diabetes Center
Affiliate at University of Maryland Medical Services
22 South Greene Street, N6W100
Baltimore, MD 21201-1595
(410) 328-6584
(888) JOSLIN-8

Joslin Diabetes Center
Affiliate at Shipley's Choice Medical Park (Satellite of University of Maryland)
8601 Veterans Highway
Millersville, MD 21108
(410) 729-4601

MASSACHUSETTS

Joslin Diabetes Center
One Joslin Place
Boston, MA 02215
(617) 732-2440

Joslin Center at Deaconess-Nashoba Hospital
220 Groton Road
Ayer, MA 01432
(978) 784-9534

Joslin Diabetes Center
Affiliate at Falmouth
210 Jones Road
Falmouth, MA 02540
(508) 548-1944

Joslin at Deaconess-Glover Hospital
148 Chestnut Street
Needham, MA 02192
(781)453-5231

Joslin Diabetes Center
Affiliate at Mercy Hospital
299 Carew Street
Springfield, MA 01104
(413) 748-7000
(877) JOSLIN-8

NEW JERSEY

Joslin Diabetes Center
Affiliate at Saint Barnabas Ambulatory Care Center
200 South Orange Avenue
Livingston, NJ 07039
(973) 322-7207

Joslin Diabetes Center
Affiliate at St. Barnabas Medical Center (Satellite of St. Barnabas)
Community Medical Center Division
368 Lakehurst Road, Suite 305
Toms River, NJ 08753
(732) 349-5757

Joslin Diabetes Center
Affiliate at Kimball Medical Center (Satellite of St. Barnabas)
600 River Avenue
Room 1050, One South
Lakewood, NJ 08701
(732) 886-4748

NEW YORK

Joslin Diabetes Center
Affiliate at SUNY Upstate Medical University
90 Presidential Plaza
Syracuse, NY 13202
(315) 464-5726

Joslin Diabetes Center
Affiliate at Hudson Valley Hospital Center
225 Veterans Road, Suite 201
Yorktown Heights, NY 10598
888-HVHC-JOSLIN ([888] 484-2567)
(914) 962-1320

Joslin Diabetes Center
Affiliate at Sound Shore Medical Center
16 Guion Place
New Rochelle, NY 10801

Joslin Diabetes Center
Affiliate at Ellenville Community Hospital
Route 209
Ellenville, NY 12428

Joslin Diabetes Center
Affiliate at Westchester Medical Center
100 Grassland Rd.
Valhalla, NY 10595

PENNSYLVANIA

Joslin Diabetes Center
Affiliate at Western Pennsylvania Hospital
5140 Liberty Avenue
Pittsburgh, PA 15224
(412) 578-1724

SOUTH CAROLINA

Joslin Diabetes Center
Affiliate at McLeod Regional Medical Center
305 East Cheves Street
Florence, SC 29506
(888) 777-6965

TENNESSEE

Joslin Diabetes Center
Affiliate at Memorial Hospital
2525 deSales Avenue
Chattanooga, TN 37404
(423) 495-7970

WASHINGTON

Joslin Diabetes Center
Affiliate at Swedish Medical Center
910 Boylston Avenue
Seattle, WA 98104-0999
(206) 215-2440
888-JOSLIN 1

WEST VIRGINIA

Joslin Diabetes Center
Affiliate at St. Mary's Hospital
2900 First Avenue
Huntington, WV 25702
(304) 526-8363

Metric Conversion Table

Liquid Measurements

¼ teaspoon = 1.25 milliliters
½ teaspoon = 2.5 milliliters
1 teaspoon = 5 milliliters
1 tablespoon = 15 milliliters
2 tablespoons = 30 milliliters
¼ cup = 60 milliliters
⅓ cup = 80 milliliters
½ cup = 120 milliliters
⅔ cup = 160 milliliters
¾ cup = 180 milliliters
1 cup = 240 milliliters
1 pint (2 cups) = 480 milliliters
1 quart (4 cups) = 960 milliliters (.96 liters)

Equivalents for Dry Measurements

AMOUNT	FINE POWDER (FLOUR)	GRAIN (RICE)
1 cup	140 grams	150 grams
¾ cup	105 grams	113 grams
⅔ cup	93 grams	100 grams
½ cup	70 grams	75 grams
⅓ cup	47 grams	50 grams
¼ cup	35 grams	38 grams
⅛ cup	18 grams	19 grams

AMOUNT	GRANULAR (SUGAR)	SOLIDS (BUTTER)
1 cup	190 grams	200 grams
¾	143 grams	150 grams
⅔ cup	125 grams	133 grams
½ cup	95 grams	100 grams
⅓ cup	63 grams	67 grams
¼ cup	48 grams	50 grams
⅛ cup	24 grams	15 grams

Oven Temperatures

	FAHRENHEIT	CELSIUS	GAS MARK
Freeze water	32°F	0°C	
Room temperature	68°F	20°C	
Boil water	212°F	100°C	
Bake	325°F	160°C	3
	350°F	180°C	4
	375°F	190°C	5
	400°F	200°C	6
	425°F	220°C	7
	450°F	230°C	8

Equivalents for Weights

1 ounce = 30 grams
4 ounces = 120 grams
8 ounces = 240 grams
12 ounces = ⅔ pound = 360 grams
16 ounces = 1 pound = 480 grams

Equivalent for Length

1 inch = 2.5 centimeters
6 inches = ½ foot = 15 centimeters
12 inches = 1 foot = 30 centimeters
36 inches = 3 feet = 1 yard = 90 centimeters
40 inches = 100 centimeters = 1 meter

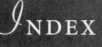

INDEX